T0133088

ADOLESCENT PSYCHIATRY

DEVELOPMENTAL AND CLINICAL STUDIES

VOLUME 23

Annals of the American Society for Adolescent Psychiatry

ADOLESCENT PSYCHIATRY

DEVELOPMENTAL AND CLINICAL STUDIES

VOLUME 23

AARON H. ESMAN

Editor in Chief

LOIS T. FLAHERTY
HARVEY A. HOROWITZ

Associate Editors

THE ANALYTIC PRESS

1998   Hillsdale, NJ   London

Published by The Analytic Press, Inc.
Editorial Offices: 101 West Street, Hillsdale, NJ 07642

ISBN 0-88163-197-3
ISSN 0226-24064-9

Printed in the United States of America
10 9 8 7 6 5 4 3 2 1

CONTENTS

IN MEMORIAM: DEREK MILLER, M.D.

AARON H. ESMAN

Derek Miller, M.D., a distinguished figure in American and international adolescent psychiatry for more than three decades, died at his home in Northbrook, Illinois, on December 26, 1997. He is survived by his wife, Doreen, their children, Jonathan, Jennifer, and Jane, and five grandchildren.

Born in Hull, England, on January 18, 1923, Dr. Miller obtained his M.B. and Ch.B. degrees at the Medical School of the University of Leeds in 1947 and an M.D. in 1955. Internships at Leeds were followed by a psychiatric residency at the Menninger Foundation in Topeka, Kansas, from 1952 to 1954, and five years as Staff Psychiatrist at that eminent institution. Returning to his native soil, he became a Senior Registrar at the Tavistock Clinic in London, where he advanced to the position of Medical Director of the Adolescent Unit, serving in that capacity until 1969; during that period, he obtained his psychoanalytic training at the Institute for Psychoanalysis in London.

In 1969, Dr. Miller returned to the United States, joining the Department of Psychiatry at the University of Michigan, Ann Arbor. There he served variously as Chief of Outpatient Adolescent Psychiatry, Chief of Adult Services, Chief of Adolescent Services, Chief of the Medical Student Mental Health Service, and, ultimately, Associate Chairman of the Department, while holding the academic rank of Clinical Professor of Psychiatry. In 1976, he moved to Chicago to become Director of the Adolescent Treatment Program at Northwestern Memorial Hospital and Professor of Psychiatry at Northwestern University. In 1991, he became the Director of the North Shore Treatment Center in Highland Park, Illinois.

A member of ASAP since 1971, Dr. Miller served as President of the Michigan Society of Adolescent Psychiatry in 1974 and was a member of the ASAP Board of Trustees and Chairman of its Membership Committee from 1974 to 1976. He was elected to Fellowship in ASAP in 1984 and became Honorary President of the International

Society for Adolescent Psychiatry in 1992. He was the recipient of a host of honors, lectureships, and visiting professorships in the United States, Europe, and South Africa.

Derek Miller was a prolific author and a major contributor to the literature in adolescent psychiatry, with a particular interest in juvenile delinquency. Profoundly committed to the medical foundations of psychiatry, his writings always emphasized both the biological and the psychosocial aspects of psychopathology and of treatment. His first book, *The Psychosocial Treatment of Delinquent Youth* (1965), a landmark work in this field, was followed by *The Age Between* (1984) and *Attack on the Self* (1986). His contributions to these *Annals* were legion, dealing with virtually every significant clinical issue in the field; his last paper, proposing improved ways of dealing with adolescents in the courts, appeared in the previous volume. He brought to his work enormous energy, therapeutic optimism, and a deeply felt empathy for the young people for whom he cared. For these characteristics, as well as for his urbanity, his wit, and his cultivated mind, he will be missed by all who knew him.

FOREWORD

REPLENISHING ASAP'S VINES: VINTAGE AND NONVINTAGE WINES

ALEX WEINTROB

As immediate past-president of the American Society for Adolescent Psychiatry (ASAP), I am very grateful to Dr. Esman for the opportunity to inform the readership of *The Annals* of the directions the Society will be taking over the next several years, into and beyond the millennium. These directions will, I believe, be reflected in the contents of *The Annals*.

It has been 40 years since the formation in New York City of the first local Society for Adolescent Psychiatry. The basic aims stated at that time were "to provide a forum for the exchange of psychiatric knowledge about the adolescent, to encourage the development of adequate training facilitates for adolescent psychiatry, to stimulate research in the psychopathology and treatment of adolescents, and to foster the development of adequate adolescent services" (Schonfeld, 1971). Over the next decade, more local societies formed and then confederated in 1967 as the American Society for Adolescent Psychiatry, whose aims reflected those of the New York Society. Four years later, *Adolescent Psychiatry* was first published, its purpose,

> to explore adolescence as a process . . . to enter challenging and exciting areas that may have profound effects on our basic concepts. . . . This volume was designed with a twofold purpose. It can stand on its own as a contribution to adolescent psychiatry. However, we hope that it will be the first volume of a series that will provide a forum for the expression of ideas and problems that plague and excite so many of us working in this enigmatic but fascinating field [Feinstein, Giovacchini, and Miller, 1971].

For many years now, both ASAP (in its annual meetings) and *The Annals* have fulfilled these stated aims, with a primary focus on psychodynamic thinking and treatment, and have acted as the leading proponents in this regard. For example, major contributors at meetings and in *The Annals* have included, to name only a very few, Anthony, Bettelheim, Blos, Ekstein, Esman, Giovacchini, Kernberg, Marohn, Masterson, Miller, Offer, Rakoff, Rinsley, and Winnicott. This psychodynamic orientation appears to be, if anything, even more important now than it was in the past to those psychiatrists currently finishing their training and entering practice. Many of us have heard complaints from these people that their training was sorely lacking in psychodynamic approaches and instead favored those short-term strategies welcomed by managed care companies. Psychiatrists new to the field have eagerly sought out presentations and articles devoted to psychodynamic thinking. Thus, ASAP is dedicated to preserving and perpetuating such thinking through our annual meetings, our Newsletter, our *Journal of Youth and Adolescence* (while currently largely a research journal, it is also dedicated to publishing clinical articles), and *The Annals* (whose editor is a major figure in psychodynamic psychiatry). Thus, the title of this Foreword, which reflects a commitment to preserving our ability to produce the highest quality vintage wines, the seminal thinking in psychodynamic adolescent psychiatry.

At the same time, it is clear that the Society must expand its horizons and play a more active role in speaking out on those issues of great concern to adolescents, their parents, and their therapists. Included among these issues (which were addressed at our last annual meeting by the presidents of all the major psychiatric associations—ASAP, the American Psychiatric Association, the Academy of Child and Adolescent Psychiatry, and the American Association of Community Psychiatrists) are:

1) Juvenile justice (in my opinion, an oxymoron in the current public and legislative views). It is becoming increasingly clear that adolescents, and particularly disturbed adolescents, are being very poorly served in the juvenile justice system. (Even this statement may be too generous. There are numerous indications that not only are mentally ill or retarded adolescents who have not committed crimes failing to receive adequate services, but also they are being subjected to punitive treatments in an atmosphere in which they are housed with those who have committed crimes.) Examples of *The Annals'* response to the overall issue are represented by the publication in Volume 22 of Kalogerakis's (1998)

address on adolescent violence at the 1997 scientific meeting and of Miller's (1998) chapter on improving psychiatric services to juvenile justice systems.

2) Psychopharmacologic treatment of adolescent disorders. It is ASAP's expectation that this issue will increasingly be addressed in our Newsletter, at our annual meetings, and in *The Annals*, perhaps with a subsection devoted to updated information regarding psychotropic medications. I believe it important to note that *The Annals* represents a marvelous venue for obtaining up-to-date information, as the time from submission to publication is shorter than it is for many scientific journals.

3) Substance use and abuse, especially nicotine, alcohol, and marijuana. This volume of *The Annals* offers a major article by Jaffe on this subject. It is clear that ASAP's members increasingly are dealing with teenagers and young adults (especially college youth) whose behaviors are adversely affected by these drugs. Recent attention has been drawn to deaths as a result of binge drinking in high schools and colleges. Our members, then, must develop the skills to address this issue both as contributors to public policy and as therapists to these young people and their families.

4) Issues regarding teenage sexuality. Note the article on AIDS by Renshaw in this volume. We can no longer sit by idly as our adolescents are engaging in high risk behaviors which often lead to disease and unwanted pregnancies.

These issues are related to my reference to nonvintage (synonymous with current, not to be cellared as with vintage) wines. We are hopeful that they will be addressed through all our various organs of communication, including *The Annals*, the *Journal of Youth and Adolescence*, the Newsletter, our annual meetings, and the work of our local societies. In addition, as we somewhat belatedly enter the new age of communication, we expect increasingly to use e-mail, an expanded database, and our soon-to-be developed web site on the Internet, the last allowing for instant communication among our members and between ASAP and the public. With our broad areas of expertise, flavored by our understanding of the adolescent process, the American Society for Adolescent Psychiatry is hopeful that through these organs we will be able to continue producing our vintage (not to be confused with old, but instead meaning excellent) psychodynamic wines as well as youthful, dynamic, and refreshing wines that address those complex current issues that plague adolescents and their families in our society.

REFERENCES

Feinstein, S. C., Giovacchini, P. & Miller, P. (1971), Preface. In: *Adolescent Psychiatry, Vol. 1*, ed. S. C. Feinstein, P. Giovacchini, & A. A. Miller. New York: Basic Books, pp. xiii–xv.

Kalogerakis, M. G. (1998), Adolescent Violence—Twentieth century madness: A critical review of theories of causation. In: *Adolescent Psychiatry, Vol. 22*, ed. A. Esman. Hillsdale, NJ: The Analytic Press, pp. 251–276.

Miller, D. (1998), Psychiatric contributions to improve the effectiveness of juvenile justice. In: *Adolescent Psychiatry, Vol. 22*, ed. A. Esman. Hillsdale, NJ: The Analytic Press, pp. 113–140.

Schonfeld, W. A. (1971), Foreword. In: *Adolescent Psychiatry, Vol. 1*, ed. S. C. Feinstein, P. Giovacchini, & A. A. Miller. New York: Basic Books, pp. vii–viii.

PART I

DEVELOPMENTAL CONSIDERATIONS

Our understanding of the adolescent process continues, as do adolescents themselves, to grow and develop with the years. New data from clinical, observational, and neurobiological sources oblige us to review, reconsider, and, when necessary, revise our notions about how the child evolves to become an adult. The late Richard Marohn, all too briefly the editor of these *Annals*, attempted such a revision of the "classical" viewpoint from the standpoint of Kohutian self psychology. Revised and edited by two of his colleagues, his essay challenges traditional views about late adolescence and the so-called second individuation process.[1] Phyllis Tyson brings together a more "classical," ego-psychological approach and recent neurobiological observations to conceptualize the impact of early problems of attachment and nurturance on the later evolution of behavior and character formation in adolescence. Steven Katz critically reviews the evidence for familial contributions to the pathogenesis of adolescent depression. Together, these chapters exemplify the continuing reassessment of familiar perspectives, which increasingly characterizes contemporary biopsychosocial views of the development of personality in general and of adolescence in particular.

[1]A symposium discussing Dr. Marohn's ideas from several perspectives will appear in Volume 24 of the *Annals*.

1   A REEXAMINATION OF PETER BLOS'S CONCEPT OF PROLONGED ADOLESCENCE

RICHARD C. MAROHN

REVISED AND EDITED BY
SHELLEY R. DOCTORS AND ROBERT J. LEIDER

The three fundamentals of psychoanalytic theory regarding adolescent development are (a) Sigmund Freud's (1905) idea of the displacement of genitality as a result of an increase in the intensity of the libidinal drive and an urgent need to defend against the incest taboo, (b) Anna Freud's (1958) description of "adolescent turmoil" and her emphasis on the loosening of infantile incestuous libidinal object ties through utilization of a variety of typical adolescent defenses, and (c) Peter Blos's concept of adolescence as a second individuation process (1967) and his theory of adolescence as a recapitulation of the oedipal period (1979).

However, despite this formidable foundation and significant modern additions and elaborations, adolescence as a developmental phase remains relatively neglected in psychoanalytic theory (A. Freud, 1958). Case reports of psychoanalytic treatment conducted in adulthood typically omit reconstructions of adolescence (Eissler, 1958). Some have attributed the genesis of the problem to the nature of adolescence itself and to the "threat" its revival presents to both analyst and analysand (e.g., Goettsche, 1986). No matter what challenges adolescent experiences and affects present to analytic technique, if analysts continue to miss the powerful impact adolescence has on the development of personality and of pathological symptoms (Beiser, 1984, p. 11), it behooves us to recognize and consider the problem.

Psychoanalytic theory has remained fascinated with the Oedipus complex because of Freud's pioneering discoveries and formulations. His emphasis on making the unconscious conscious and on recovering repressed childhood memories led most psychoanalytic work to focus on early childhood. However, recent reformulations of psychoanalytic theory derived from an increased emphasis on the data of infant observation and on the findings of self psychology have enabled us to view the developmental process differently and thus provide us with a new perspective from which to view adolescence.

My focus here is on the concept of "prolonged adolescence." This notion—of a particular kind of adolescent pathology—is based on the classical view of adolescence as a reworking of the oedipal period. It is my view that placing the Oedipus complex at the center of adolescence—continuing to see the relational shifts of the period as primarily related to the Oedipus complex—skews our understanding of adolescence in the lives of all our patients. I believe it causes us to see certain young adults as sick, and it blinds us to the healthy aspects of our patients. I hope to advance the idea that a view of adolescence based on self-psychological understandings avoids the pitfalls associated with the theory of prolonged adolescence and allows an enhanced understanding of adolescent and adult patients.

Prolonged Adolescence

Prolonged adolescence[1] was first described by Siegfried Bernfeld (1923) in a presentation to the Vienna Psychoanalytic Society on February 15, 1922.[2] Bernfeld sketched a group of male adolescents whose psychical desire for an object extended beyond the physiological process of genital drive. He described certain characteristics and distinguished "this complex . . . from the definition of puberty as given by Freud" (in Jones, 1925, p. 478).

These youths become preoccupied with ideals and aesthetics; they become painfully depressed trying to produce a work of art, a new form of politics, or some similar humanistic endeavor; and, further, in these youths, "the sexual components do not concentrate on finding

---

[1]Bernfeld's term was adopted by Blos (1954) and by A. Freud (1958). Bernfeld's original meaning may have been altered as the term became popularized.

[2]The original has not been translated from German. Those reading only English are limited to the abstract that appears in the *International Journal of Psycho-Analysis* (Jones, 1925).

an object, a great part is turned into ego-libido, creating thus a new (secondary) narcissistic situation" (Bernfeld, in Jones, 1925, pp. 477–478). Bernfeld referred several times to these characteristics as adolescent narcissistic transformations that cannot be reduced to archaic fixations or regressions, and he did not characterize those youths as disturbed.

When Peter Blos (1979)[3] wrote about "prolonged male adolescence," he noted that Bernfeld had investigated the "social phenomenon observed in European youth movements after the First World War" (p. 38). Blos continued, "Members of these groups presented a strong predilection for intellectualization and sexual repression, thus delaying the resolution of the adolescent conflict, and in consequence, the personality consolidation of late adolescence (p. 38)."[4,5]

In a commentary, Anna Freud (1958) summarized Bernfeld's "protracted type" of male adolescence as follows: "[It] extends far beyond the time limit normal for adolescent characteristics, and is conspicuous by tendencies toward productivity whether artistic, literary or scientific, and by a strong bent toward idealistic aims and spiritual values" (p. 257); and she continued, "Bernfeld accounted in this manner for the elaborations of the normal adolescent processes by the impact of internal frustrations and external, environmental pressures" (p. 257).

For Blos (1954), the term *prolonged adolescence* had begun to lose specificity, and so he described his subject quite precisely: "the American middle-class young man, roughly between eighteen and twenty-two, who usually attends college or has, at any rate, some professional aspirations; this fact, more often than not, makes him financially dependent on his family during the years of early adulthood" (pp. 733–734). Blos (1979) maintained that the configuration he had described in 1954 was still valid (p. 38, footnote 1), and he added that this was so, even though the phenomenology had changed radically in

---

[3]Blos's influential paper was first published in 1954. An edited and slightly revised version was published in 1979. The changes made in the 1979 paper were primarily stylistic rather than substantive. In Dr. Marohn's preliminary manuscript, some quotations used the wording of the 1954 version, others that of the 1979 version. In a few citations, we have indicated the wording of each version.

[4]This characterization may represent Blos's formulation. It may not be true to Bernfeld's original presentation.

[5]Blos's original statement (1954, p. 733) is identical except for the phrase, "and, in consequence, the personality consolidation of late adolescence," which was added in 1979.

the intervening 25 years (society now had *dropout* and *alternative life styles*) and despite the general acceptance of Erikson's concept of a "psychosocial moratorium."

Blos (1954) defined prolonged adolescence as:

a static perseveration in the adolescent position which under normal circumstances is of a time-limited and transitory nature. A developmental phase which is intended to be left behind after it has accomplished its task has become a way of life. Instead of the progressive push, which normally carries the adolescent into adulthood, prolonged adolescence arrests this forward motion with the result that the adolescent process is not abandoned but kept open indefinitely. In fact, the adolescent crisis is adhered to with persistence, desperation, and anxiousness. . . . The fervent clinging to the unsettledness of all of life's issues renders any progression to adulthood an achievement which is hardly worth the price. This dilemma leads to the contrivance of ingenious ways to combine childhood gratifications with adult prerogatives. The adolescent strives to bypass the finality of choices and options exacted at the close of adolescence [p. 734].

Blos continued:

The essential difference which sets off the cases under consideration from other forms of adolescent reaction . . . seems to lie in a remarkable resistivity against the regressive pull in conjunction with a persistent avoidance of any consolidation of the adolescent process . . . prolonged adolescence is the expression of an inner necessity to keep the adolescent crisis open [p. 735].

The adolescent process can be considered closed when a hierarchical and relatively inflexible organization of genital and pregenital drives has been attained, and when ego functions have acquired a significant resistivity to regression. . . . In sharp contrast to the ego-differentiating processes that are typical for adolescent character synthesis, prolonged adolescence is characterized by a failure to arrive at a stable, indeed inflexible, hierarchical organization of drives and ego functions [1979, p. 43[6]]. . . . When these adoles-

---

[6]In 1954, the last line read as follows: "In sharp contrast to ego-differentiating processes which are so typical for adolescent synthesis, it appears that prolonged

cents attempt the rupture of their childhood dependencies, they soon realize that this move is accompanied by a narcissistic impoverishment for which they are not prepared and which they cannot tolerate [1979, p. 45[7]].

Here Blos described prolonged adolescence as similar to a character disorder: The changes are not experienced as ego-alien. But, as is not the case with a character disorder, there is no rigidity, there is flexibility, adolescent flexibility—for a time. "Eventually—in the early or middle twenties—prolonged adolescence yields to a more organized and rigid settlement; the narcissistic character disorder describes best the general trend of the pathological development prolonged adolescence will take" (Blos, 1979, p. 49).[8]

Blos's view of adolescence (based on the drive model modified, to some extent, by ego psychology and object relations theory) relies heavily on Mahler's (Mahler, Pine, and Bergman, 1975) work on separation-individuation. This model, which focuses on genitality and autonomy, cannot account for the men described, who continue to work on narcissistic transformations that utilize both original and new selfobjects. Hence, when encountered, they are labeled a *pathological variant*. I think that, by confusing "inflexibility" and "resistivity to regression" with stability and health, Blos missed the variations found in each self's compensatory structures.

The Prevalent View of Adolescence

Although Erikson (1968) built his psychology of adaptation on the foundations of traditional drive theory, he noted that "libido theo-

---

adolescence is characterized by a failure at the hierarchical organization of drives and ego functions" (p. 736).

[7]In 1954, this was expressed in two sentences: "This is precisely what happens when these adolescents attempt the rupture of their emotional ties. They suddenly realize that this move is accompanied by a narcissistic impoverishment which they are unable to tolerate" (p. 737).

[8]In 1954, the language is identical except that an additional word, "finally," is included, and the last phrase reads: "the general trend of the pathological development which prolonged adolescence will finally take" (p. 739).

ry . . . offers no adequate account . . . for . . . prolonged adolescence. Here the sexually matured individual is more or less retarded in his psychosexual capacity for intimacy and in the psychosocial readiness for parenthood" (p. 156). In order to explain this phenomenon, Erikson introduced the concept of a psychosocial moratorium—a period in which society permits a latency or delay of psychosexual development to allow for role experimentation in the service of consolidation of previous achievements and of new identities. I believe that he postulated a "moratorium" in order to account for the discrepancy between his observations of adolescent development and those expected by the prevailing theory (the model of the progression of separation-individuation and structural closure) and also to make sure that he was not misunderstood and thought to be speaking of that pathological state, prolonged adolescence.

As Singer (1987) observed, the use of the separation-individuation model persists in the theories and practices of many influential contemporary adolescent clinicians. For example, when Masterson (1980) refers to individuation and independence, he seems committed to the developmental model of adolescent separation-individuation. Similarly, despite the fact that Offer challenged the traditional models of adolescent development and pathology (specifically the idea that "adolescent turmoil" is normative), he and Baittle (Baittle and Offer, 1971) adhered to the traditional model of separation-individuation when they wrote that "the main function of rebellion in the normal adolescent is . . . to initiate or reinforce a process that leads to emancipation from the parents" (p. 152).

Dissenters from the Separation-Individuation Model of Adolescence

Roy Schafer (1973) challenged the term *separation-individuation* as a concretism, a manifestation of primary-process thinking, which, like *detachment* and similar terms, are at best metaphors, not actualities. Schafer is "opposed to the use of the term 'individuation' in connection with adolescence, because it further complicates rather than deepens our understanding of this phase" (p. 45), and he implies that, in individuating, one does not give up ties to infantile object representations:

Genuine emancipation seems to be built on revision, modulation, and selective acceptance as well as rejection, flexible mastery, and complex substitutions and other changes of aims, representations, and patterns of behavior. These changes are necessarily slow, subtle, ambivalent, limited, and fluctuating [p. 45].

Many others have taken issue with Blos's conception of adolescence as eventuating in a final consolidation and structuralization of the personality. For example, Escoll (1987) wrote, "Often the consolidation we expect to find exists more as a patch quilt. . . . We might describe many young adults as on the way to consolidation, with consolidation being seen at different stages of resolution and not firmly achieved until later on, sometimes only well into the late young-adult or adult years" (p. 10).

Galatzer-Levy (1984) contends that, even though Blos's view (that the termination of normal adolescence involves thorough renunciation of object-libidinal and nondrive needs toward the parents) has little clinical support, it is well entrenched in the ideas of Freud, Mahler, and Western philosophy. In fact, Galatzer-Levy quotes Anthony and Benedek (1970) and Cohler and Grunebaum (1980) in claiming that "long-term engagements with parents and grandparents, both on a manifest and a deep psychological level, are an aspect of the healthy development of many children and parents" (p. 45).

Kenny (1987), in a study of 173 first-year college students, challenged the view that healthy autonomy requires the loosening of family ties. He found that, among securely attached (Ainsworth et al., 1978) college students, "most students viewed their parents as a secure base, encouraging independence and remaining available as a source of support when needed" (p. 17). Curiously, Kenny reported that feelings of closeness to parents usually increase following departure from a family—indicating, perhaps, that the attachment remains important throughout the process of leaving home and may continue to function as a healthy support.

The Route to Self Psychology

Maxwell Gitelson, who may have significantly influenced Kohut, emphasized as early as 1942 that an empathic relationship is crucial in producing therapeutic change in adolescence. Gitelson believed that the therapist needed to make and maintain "narcissistic contact" with the patient. He spoke of this bond much as we now speak of the self–selfobject bond—as sustaining patients through hard times—and he described the therapeutic task in adolescents as one of "character synthesis" (Gitelson, 1948).

In my opinion (Marohn, 1980), ideas about narcissistic bonding are more useful in understanding the struggles of the adolescent to separate from infantile attachments to parents than is the usual emphasis on libidinal incestuous attachments. As young people mature, they separate psychologically from the parents of childhood by achieving a different sense of the relationship: Parents are no longer slavishly idolized or adored but remain as respected, important, valued human beings in one's life (Marohn, 1984). Adolescents defend against their childhood attachments by de-idealization and disparagement, by negating mirroring, and by stimulating disgust. They displace their needs for narcissistic bonds onto peers or onto other adults and thus develop crushes, infatuations, and other varieties of self–selfobject connection.

Much delinquent behavior can be best understood as a manifestation of primitive narcissism (Marohn, 1977; Marohn et al., 1979; Offer, Marohn, and Ostrov, 1979). Sociopathy and antisocial behavior are not correctly understood when thought to result from a deficient superego; rather, they result from difficulties in self-esteem regulation and the primitive use of selfobjects. Similarly, as self-regulation and affect regulation may for some adolescents be difficult developmental tasks, substance abuse in adolescents is often found to result from difficulties in self-soothing. And impulsive adolescents behave violently and assault other patients or staff because they are traumatically overstimulated by affectionate longings, not because of a destructive aggressive drive (Marohn et al., 1973; Marohn, 1974). They are pessimistic about the future because of an awareness of the inadequacy of their self-regulation, not because of strong internalized punitive superego attitudes (Marohn, 1971). These are narcissistic problems, not moral difficulties or deficiencies!

Many mental health professionals unfortunately respond to such negativism in adolescents by avoiding them—especially impulsive or delinquent adolescents. Because of their size and their greater propensity for violence, such adolescents are often shunted into the juvenile justice and correctional systems, whereas earlier, as children, they had been seen in child psychiatry facilities (Marohn, 1981).

My own experience in working therapeutically with disturbed adolescents in both hospital and office settings is more positive. It led me, and my colleagues, to formulate a variety of empirically based, eclectic, clinical theories and treatment interventions. In the hospital milieu, the staff and structure of the treatment program provide important selfobject functions needed to buttress the patient's self-regulation and to facilitate the psychotherapy process (Marohn et al., 1980). The therapist's use of his or her own self as a confident individual provides the adolescent with a secure selfobject (a person who does not need to be mirrored or idealized by the adolescent) who does not need to stimulate the adolescent or become the focus of an idealizing transference. Such a therapist can be effective in promoting psychological development and therapeutic change.

Psychology of the Self

Today, self psychology, rather than being viewed as an alternative paradigm to traditional drive theory, has begun to refashion much of clinical practice. The significance of the empathic vantage point in effecting sound treatment (and the centrality of the paradigm of the self–selfobject dyad) is increasingly recognized. Flexibility and personality enrichment in the "area of progressive neutralization" (Kohut and Seitz, 1978) achieve new importance in a reconsideration of adolescent development.

Adolescence brings with it a reworking of the internal experience of the relationship between the self and its selfobjects—not that this is the first revision since the oedipal age, for fundamental to the self–selfobject model is the recognition that the dyad is continually moving toward redefinition. However, adolescence is a phase of marked and dramatic transformation. The healthy self modifies and adjusts the nature and meaning of the relationship between itself and its selfobjects consistent with ongoing physiological and cognitive development. Yet, it maintains enriching ties with the archaic selfobjects—the parents of infancy and childhood.

Thus, adolescence does not involve a separation from the "infantile incestuous objects" (or their representations) and individuation but, rather (in language borrowed from Schafer), modifications, shifts, changes, revisions, variations, and transformations in the nature of their

11

relationship. To be truly psychoanalytic, we look not at the social, external, or physical relationship (e.g., does the daughter live at home or away; does she call home frequently); instead, we assess the nature of the inner experience (e.g., does the internal representation of her mother sustain her; does she reexperience such sustenance in new relationships with teachers, boyfriends, or others). She has not psychologically separated from her mother and become an autonomous individual with no further tie to mother; rather, she has built on that tie, modified that bond, and calls on it regularly to serve as a template from which to forge and shape new relationships while preserving aspects of the old.

As Palombo (1987) stressed, the adolescent's needs for selfobjects are quite different from those of previous developmental stages. They are certainly not a simple recapitulation of earlier needs.

> Adolescents arrive at this phase with specific developmental needs for particular responses from their caretakers. The nature of the selfobject functions required at this stage is different from those of prior stages. . . . While adolescents may bring with them unresolved issues or selfobject deficits from prior developmental stages, these only serve to render more complex the task of the traversal of this phase. These deficits, or the regressions to prior modes of functioning, do not constitute the essence of the phase-appropriate struggle. Rather the complementing of the self by new selfobject functions is central to the negotiation of this phase [p. 175].

What, then, can we say about the clinical phenomena Blos and others have described and frequently witnessed? They were sound clinicians who attempted to explain the increased development of well-functioning psychological structures in the adolescent. But, they considered them to be replacements for, and outgrowths of, relationships with the primary objects—the parents.[9]

---

[9]Wolf (1982) commented that, in 1972, he and his colleagues held a similar view. That is, to paraphrase Wolf, they—still influenced by the model of an ego striving for independence, self-sufficiency, and autonomy—thought that the adolescent's need for selfobject function would diminish and eventually be discarded.

We now recognize that these seemingly autonomous structures do not replace the archaic selfobjects; rather, they represent shifts in the relationships with these selfobjects—that is, the development of more mature selfobject relationships with the selfobjects of childhood. As the gaze and smile replace the hug and cuddle, the father's words to the adolescent and his ideals supplant the roughhousing and playing catch of the latency period. Perhaps the 20-year-old can now soothe and comfort himself, whereas earlier he required the solace of mother. Later, he experimented with friendships and substances to derive a different kind of soothing. But, all along, the effectiveness of that soothing, other or self, builds on the nature and evolution of the archaic bonds. The healthy 20-year-old gains sustenance from memories of comfort and relief and even more from the imperceptible effects such experiences have on the personality and character. Clearly, his ability to perform these functions himself has not replaced others' doing it for him, but these functions now rely on new and different selfobject ties that mirror him in a different way, serve as ideals for further psychological growth, and support his psychological cohesion.

What, then, are the goals of adolescence? And, if adolescence is assumed to have an endpoint, how may that be defined? Wolf reiterated a point made often by Kohut (1977, 1984)—that the self never gives up its need for selfobjects; rather, with increasing consolidation of the self, the intensity and form of the selfobject needs change. As Wolf (1982) stated, "The self's goals are not autonomy and independence but cohesiveness in its striving for integration into a reciprocally responsive matrix of selfobject relationships" (p. 179). By way of example, Wolf noted the adolescent's decreasing need for the peer group. He commented that this is not due to a decreased need for a selfobject relationship but occurs because of changes in selfobject needs: Maturation of the self and maturation of cognitive capacity now allow for the construction of symbolic selfobjects. Palombo (1987) spoke in a similar vein. He too considered that adolescence culminated in the consolidation of the self.

Wolf (1982) and Palombo (1987) both speak of adolescence ending when the young adult has chosen the vocation, companions, and avenues through which he will express his values and ideals.[10] Those who (from

---

[10]Wolf (1982), however, noted that development does not come to an end with adolescence, or when maturity is said to be reached.

a social point of view) remain unable to effect such choices fall into prolonged adolescence as described by Blos. However, from the self-psychological perspective, the process of adolescent development is not one of renouncing infantile incestuous object ties. Thus, we understand the underlying, unconscious causes of prolonged adolescence very differently than does Blos.

The critical issue is that the classical drive model and its later derivatives in ego psychology present us with a view of drives to be tamed, primitive urges to be renounced, and autonomous functioning to be achieved by late adolescence. The self-psychological model shifts attention and focus from separation-individuation to the changes, modifications, and differences in the experience of the self with its selfobjects. These attachments are not replaced—they are changed, altered, and refashioned. These attachments evolve and support, rather than replace, psychological functions. This is the essence of the transmuting internalizations achieved in healthy adolescent development and in successful treatment.[11]

The self–selfobject paradigm has shifted the focus of psychoanalysis by emphasizing the importance of the self–selfobject dyad and of the selfobject experience. The selfobject relationship is transformed over the life span. Selfobjects are not given up at the close of adolescence. The continued use of selfobjects is an integral part of adulthood.

Discussion

Prolonged adolescence is not a psychopathological state but the result of inadequate theory applied to reliable data. If one sees adolescence as ushered in by an increase in libidinal drive (S. Freud, 1905), and the concomitant developmental task as that of the loosening of infantile incestuous object ties (A. Freud, 1958), then the separation-individuation paradigm follows. That view of adolescence (as a recapitulation of separation-individuation) states that continued psychological contact with the "infantile objects" is evidence of immaturity. The self–

---

[11]Marohn was well aware of criticisms of self psychology. The original manuscript of this paper (of which this is an edited and condensed rendering) contained a lengthy section addressing those (e.g., Greenberg and Mitchell, 1983) who fault self psychology as merely using new terms to restate old concepts.

selfobject paradigm offers an alternative—that, throughout adolescence and adulthood, one retains ties to selfobjects. One never separates, individuates, or becomes psychologically independent. One remains psychologically connected. The contrast between these models is dramatic!

Traditional theory tells us that adolescents should separate and individuate—that they should "give up" childhood claims and "grow up." Yet, somehow patients, friends, children, and research subjects don't behave that way. This bias has permeated much of our culture and much of psychoanalytic thinking, and it may be responsible for much of the normative "turmoil" described in the literature. Adolescents are uneasy because they believe they should be "breaking" their ties to their parents—and they are not disposed to do so.

To equate adolescence with giving up the incestuous objects of infancy implies that one moves from Point 1 to Point 2 without having gone through gradual shifts in the self–selfobject relationship—1.1, 1.2, 1.3, 1.x,. . . . No one really believes that, except those who see nothing happening in latency and see adolescence as simply a reworking of the oedipal period. Must we continue to hold to a model that does not capture the gradual and flexible shifts that occur in healthy adolescence? Must we continue to hold to a model that suggests an all-or-nothing breach in adolescents' relationships with their parents? Although we all know it's not that way, we continue to embrace a theory that implies it is. Why?

As the new findings of infant research question or negate many of the traditional teachings of the drive model, so does a great deal of clinical and research work with adolescents demand that we separate from the individuation model. We can build on those models while recognizing how some adolescents are crippled because they are unable to maintain sustaining ties with their parents.

The new model speaks of gradual shifts in the self–selfobject relationship as experienced intrapsychically (viz., self–selfobject 1.0 → self–selfobject 1.1 → self–selfobject 1.2, etc). Certainly, A. Freud (1958) had this in mind when she spoke of displacement of libidinal attachments onto peers and when she noted that the healthy adolescent is the flexible, experimenting one, the one who separates in a gradual, stepwise fashion. However, her theory needed, in addition, some sense of regulatory structure that organizes and guides the gradual displacements she described. We now recognize that the gradual investment in new selfobjects (peers, other adults, heroes, fictional characters, sexual partners) occurs within the context of the original, archaic self–selfobject tie, as modified and transformed in the preceding preadolescent years. It is, in fact, the sustenance of the parents, as experienced by the adolescent, that facilitates the gradual investment of new relationships.

Conclusion

The adolescent phase is neglected in case reports because accepted traditional theory does not adequately illuminate inner psychological life as revealed in psychoanalytic treatment. I claim that, contrary to the traditional psychoanalytic view, the psychology of adolescence does not emanate from the vicissitudes of genitality. Adolescence is not primarily a reworking of the Oedipus complex. The emphasis on giving up unconscious infantile incestuous libidinal objects and, more generally, on a recapitulation of separation-individuation, though theoretically elegant, does not correctly describe the adolescent process. If we continue to believe that it does, we will see adolescents as sick who aren't—as in prolonged adolescence. Further, to continue to hold that successful adolescent development must eventuate in a relatively inflexible organization of drives and defenses blinds us to healthy manifestations of the adolescent period and to the continuous nature of development in adulthood.

The value of self psychology lies in its emphasis on the personal experience in the clinical situation; in its view that introspection and empathy define the depth-psychological field; and on its willingness to modify theory when necessary, even at the expense of time-honored doctrine. Prolonged adolescence is a restatement of the idea that the closure of adolescence and initiation of young adulthood involve renunciation of ties to parents and establishment of an inflexible character structure—truly autonomous, fully individuated, and completely separated.

Just as the transference persists after the termination of an analysis, so does the evolving tie to our selfobjects persist beyond adolescence. There is no final closure at the end of adolescence. Transmuting internalization, structuralization, and the traits of empathy, wisdom, and creativity come gradually. It is the openness of the adolescent self–selfobject equation that promises an adult who is open to new ideas, who welcomes new experience, and who is yet invigorated by reaching back into the archaic past.

Let us no longer speak of adolescent separation and individuation! Let us speak, as Wolf, Gedo, and Terman (1972) did many years ago, of adolescence as a significant period in the "transformation of the self." And let us recognize that the process of developmental transformation continues into adulthood.

So it is that adolescence is "prolonged."

REFERENCES

Ainsworth, M., Blehar, M., Walters, E. & Wally, S. (1978), *Patterns of Attachment: A Psychological Study of the Strange Situation.* Hillsdale, NJ: Lawrence Erlbaum Associates, Inc.

Anthony, J. & Benedek, T. (1970), *Parenthood: Its Psychology and Psychopathology.* New York: Little Brown.

Baittle, B. & Offer, D. (1971), On the nature of male adolescent rebellion. *Adoles. Psychiat.,* 1:139–160.

Beiser, H. R. (1984), An example of self analysis. *J. Amer. Psychoanal. Assn.,* 32:3–12.

Bernfeld, S. (1923), Uber eine typische Form der mannlichen Pubertat [On a typical model of male puberty]. *Imago,* 9:169–188.

Blos, P. (1954), Prolonged male adolescence: The formulation of a syndrome and its therapeutic implications. *Amer. J. Orthopsych.,* 24:733–742.

———— (1967), The second individuation process of adolescence. *The Psychoanalytic Study of the Child,* 22:162–186. New York: International Universities Press.

———— (1979), *The Adolescent Passage.* Madison, CT: International Universities Press.

Cohler, B. & Grunebaum, H. (1980), *Grandmothers, Mothers, Daughters.* New York: Wiley.

Eissler, K. (1958), Notes on problems of technique in the psychoanalytic treatment of adolescents. *The Psychoanalytic Study of the Child,* 13:223–254. New York: International Universities Press.

Erikson, E. H. (1968), *Identity, Youth and Crisis.* New York: Norton.

Escoll, P. (1987), The psychoanalysis of young adults. *Psychoanal. Inq.,* 7:5–30.

Freud, A. (1958), Adolescence. *The Psychoanalytic Study of the Child,* 13:255–278. New York: International Universities Press.

17

Freud, S. (1905), *Three essays on the theory of sexuality. Standard Edition*, 7:130–243. London: Hogarth Press, 1953.

Galatzer-Levy, R. (1984), Adolescent breakdown and middle-age crises. In: *Late Adolescence, Psychoanalytic Studies*, ed. D. D. Brockman. New York: International Universities Press, pp. 29–51.

Gitelson, M. (1942), Direct psychotherapy in adolescence. The 1941 symposium: Case presentation by Dr. Maxwell Gitelson. *Amer. J. Orthopsychiat.*, 12:1–41.

———— (1948), Character synthesis: The psychotherapeutic problem of adolescence. *Amer. J. Orthopsychiat.*, 18:422–431.

Goettsche, R. (1986), Reconstruction of adolescence in adult analysis. *The Psychoanalytic Study of the Child*, 41:357–377. New Haven, CT: Yale University Press.

Greenberg, J. & Mitchell, S. (1983), *Object Relations in Psychoanalytic Theory*. Cambridge, MA: Harvard University Press.

Jones, K. (1925), Abstracts/Sexuality, *Inter. J. Psycho-Anal.*, 6:477–478.

Kenny, M. (1987), The extent and function of parental attachment among first-year college students. *J. Youth & Adoles.*, 16:17–29.

Kohut, H. (1977), *The Restoration of the Self*. New York, International Universities Press.

———— (1984), *How Does Analysis Cure?* ed. A. Goldberg & P. Stepansky. Chicago: University of Chicago Press.

———— & Seitz, P. (1978), Concepts and theories of psychoanalysis. In: *Concepts of Personality*, ed. J. M. Wepman & R. Heine. Chicago: Aldine, pp. 113–141.

Mahler, M. S., Pine, F. & Bergman, A. (1975), *The Psychological Birth of the Human Infant*. New York: Basic Books.

Marohn, R. (1971), Juvenile delinquents view their impulsivity. *Amer. J. Psychiat.*, 128:418–423.

———— (1974), Trauma and the delinquent. *Adoles. Psychiat.*, 3:354–361.

———— (1977), The "juvenile imposter": Some thoughts on narcissism and the delinquent. *Adoles. Psychiat.*, 5:186–212. Chicago: University of Chicago Press.

———— (1980), Adolescent rebellion and the task of separation. *Adoles. Psychiat.*, 8:173–183.

———— (1981), The negative transference in the treatment of juvenile delinquents. *The Annual of Psychoanalysis*, 11:21–42. New York: International Universities Press.

———— (1984), Disappointing and deviant youth and the rage of the elders. *Children & Youth Services Rev.*, 6:367–373.

———— Dalle-Molle, D., McCarter, E. & Linn, D. (1980), *Juvenile Delinquents—Psychodynamic Assessment and Hospital Treatment*. New York: Brunner/Mazel.

———— Dalle-Molle, D., Offer, D. & Ostrov, E. (1973), A hospital riot: Its determinants and implications for treatment. *Amer. J. Psychiat.*, 130:631–636.

———— Offer, D., Ostrow, E. & Trujullo, J. (1979), Four psychodynamic types of hospitalized juvenile delinquents. *Adoles. Psychiat.*, 7:466–483.

Offer, D, Marohn, R. C. & Ostrow, E. (1979), *The Psychological World of the Juvenile Delinquent*. New York: Basic Books.

Palombo, J. (1987), Adolescent development, A view from self psychology. *Child & Adoles. Soc. Work J.*, 5:171–186.

Schafer, R. (1973), Concepts of self and identity and the experience of separation-individuation in adolescence. *Psychoanal. Quart.*, 42:42–59.

Singer, M. (1987), A phenomenology of the self: Appersonalization, a subcategory of borderline pathology. *Psychoanal. Inq.*, 7:121–137.

Wolf, E. (1982), Adolescence: Psychology of the self and selfobjects. *Adoles. Psychiat.*, 10:171–181.

———— Gedo, J. & Terman, D. (1972), On the adolescent process as a transformation of the self. *J. Youth & Adoles.*, 1:257–272.

19

DEVELOPMENTAL ROOTS

       OF ADOLESCENT DISTURBANCE

PHYLLIS TYSON

On May 9, 1967, the American Society for Adolescent Psychiatry
was formed under the leadership of William A. Schonfeld, Sheldon
Selesnick, Sherman Feinstein, and Herman Staples. They recognized
that adolescence is "a period in which experiences have far-reaching
consequences in the synthesis and stabilization of character formation"
(Feinstein, Giovacchini, and Miller, 1971, p. xiv). "The basic aims of
the Society were to provide a forum for the exchange of psychiatric
knowledge about the adolescent, to encourage the development of
adequate training facilities for adolescent psychiatry, to stimulate research in the psychopathology and treatment of adolescents, and to
foster the development of adequate adolescent services" (p. vii). The
first scientific meetings were conducted in 1969 and 1970, and, in
1971, the first of what became an annual series "to explore adolescence
as a process" (p. xiv) was published under the editorship of Sherman
Feinstein, Peter Giovacchini, and Arthur Miller. Feinstein remained
devoted to this project, and, under his leadership, 19 volumes were
published. It is indeed an honor to offer this lecture in his memory.
    In the preface to the first volume, the editors recognized that adoles-
cent behavior, moratoriums, and other actions might be seen as adaptations designed to achieve characterological stability. So often the
adolescent suffers from "general adjustment difficulties rather than
discrete symptoms" and is "not so easily conceptualized in a psychodynamic frame of intrapsychic conflicts, but is more easily understood
in ego-psychological or behavioral terms with the sources of the tensions
in adolescence itself," although "infantile factors continue exerting their
effects" (Feinstein et al., 1971, p. xiv).
    Peter Blos, whom we also honor at this meeting, wrote the first
chapter in the first volume of *Adolescent Psychiatry*. He had only

recently (1967) published his first paper on the second individuation process—a paper that became the foundation for important subsequent work that provides the basis of our current psychoanalytic understanding of the adolescent process. Standing on the shoulders of these two giants, I have chosen to build on the notion set out in the first volume—that is, that adolescent suffering often has as its sources the tensions of the adolescent process itself. Knowing what we now know about the challenges of that process, largely due to Blos, we recognize that labile affects, heightened anxiety, and mood swings are particularly characteristic of adolescence. Recognizing that "infantile factors continue exerting their effects," I have chosen to focus this paper on affect regulation and its developmental roots. I recognize that this subject is vast, with many interrelated genetic, environmental, and neurobiological as well as psychological contributors. My focus is primarily on the psychological, with the hope that, with better understanding of early development, we might better understand those adolescents who are unable to adaptively weather the affective storms of adolescence as they negotiate the second individuation process. I begin with three short clinical vignettes to focus this discussion.

At 17, Karen was depressed and wished she would die. She and her boyfriend of 2 years had just broken up. It had been a roller-coaster relationship, and she knew he was wrong for her, but she couldn't bring herself to leave him. He was abusive and treated her like dirt, her friends told her. He insulted her in front of her friends, got mad if she didn't spend every minute of her lunch hour with him, often caused her to be late to class or to be so upset that she couldn't concentrate anyway, and her grades had begun to plummet. She thought sex was wrong, it should be saved for marriage, and she hated herself because she hadn't been strong enough to say "no" to her boyfriend. But she didn't want him to be mad at her or to dump her. When he was nice, he could be so loving, so much fun, and funny and creative. But, then he could turn on her and become so rageful. Her parents made her break up. They just didn't understand. She hates them. The boyfriend seemed to get another girlfriend so easily. He's probably having sex with her, and probably everybody knows what a slut she is. She feels terrible. She and her mother are in a constant state of war.

Sixteen-year-old Greta said she was happy now that she's run away from home to live with her boyfriend. She could not get along with her mother and step-father. Every minute at home was hell. They did this and that, this and that—it was their fault she ran away, them and their stupid rules. Grades—the teachers are so stupid. Drugs? Well—why not, all her friends do them, parties can be so boring without them. Sex—she feels lonely when she does not have a boyfriend. She's been sexually active since she was 13 and has had many boyfriends. This one is special, though. She knows he loves her. She knows she is pregnant, but she does not want an abortion. Did she have any problems? No, not really, just her stupid parents.

Tom, a 15-year-old, was oppositional and defiant at home and at school. His academic performance was declining, and he had withdrawn from social activities. Although described by his parents as a challenging child, Tom's oppositionalism and defiance became especially evident at age 13, when he began seventh grade. He did well academically, but he verbally battled with his teacher and parents. He frequently complained of a fever or stomach upset to avoid school. By the end of eighth grade, he was turning in few assignments, and his grades had plummeted. He was kicked off his soccer team due to defiance and hostility toward the coach, he had stopped participating in karate, and he was asked to leave his carpool group. Soon after beginning ninth grade, several notes that Tom had written to his 13-year-old girlfriend were confiscated by her mother. These were judged to contain sexual and suicidal overtones, and Tom was suspended from school due to "sexual harassment." Tom says these difficulties are due to his father's overcontrol and others' inability to understand him. For example, Tom shouted obscenities at his father because father had angrily pulled out the power plug on Tom's computer when he was slow to take out the trash. He wishes everyone would just leave him alone. He admits using marijuana from time to time but denies any ongoing substance abuse.

Sturm und Drang? Maybe not on the outside for all adolescents, and maybe not particularly "noisy" for all. But adolescence is a time of inner flux and change, as certain psychological tasks must be accomplished for successful adult adaptation. The adolescent must own and master adult sexuality along with an adult body. The adolescent must separate from and become independent of not only the parents of the present but also the parents of the past. This means giving up old hurts and grudges, old idealizations of the wished-for parents. Adolescents must also give up their parents as the ultimate voice of wisdom and authority; this means taking responsibility for themselves and their actions. Blos (1967) has called our attention to the challenges posed by these tasks by labeling the process the *second individuation*. He uses that label because the conflicts, related affects, and necessary tasks are reminiscent of the early-childhood process Mahler (Mahler, Pine, and Bergman, 1975) characterized as *separation-individuation.* The importance of the individual's completing this process in order to achieve characterological stability remains underappreciated. But, I believe that many of the adjustment problems we see in our adult patients—failure to achieve job stability, failed relationships, failed marriages—stem from failure to complete the tasks of the second individuation of adolescence.

For the adolescent to accomplish these tasks, new adaptations are called for; making new adaptations leads to inner flux and change. Changes made in one area shift the previous psychological balance so that other changes are needed. These in turn call for yet additional change. Intense anxiety and fear as well as excitement accompany this inner flux and change. A young person's success or lack thereof in coping with the stress and anxiety brought by these shifts and changes may be determined to a large extent by the kinds of psychological tools accrued before the hormonal changes of puberty begin to occur.

Theoretical Approaches

Although labile affects, heightened anxiety, and mood swings are particularly characteristic of adolescence, not all adolescents manifest the kinds of disturbance illustrated by Karen, Greta, and Tom. Some become stars of the football team, champion students. Some negotiate with their parents a balance between reasonable rules and independence and look forward to the time they can set their own rules; they recognize that some situations make them anxious, but they also recognize this before they become overwhelmed, and they try to understand why, seek solace from a friend, or go shoot a few baskets.

Why is it that some adolescents are able to cope with the anxiety and challenge of adolescence and accomplish its necessary tasks while maintaining relative psychic equilibrium, whereas others come to grief over the task? They become overwhelmed with the *Sturm und Drang.*

Psychoanalysts have historically approached the question of affect regulation by studying the functioning of the mind. Freud proposed a hypothetical self-regulatory psychological system he called *ego,* normally experienced as a sense of self. This system functioned to organize and regulate the individual's adaptation to the inner and outer worlds.

Disturbing affects, anxiety in particular, he associated with conflict and danger, and he suggested that they could function in one of two ways. Affects could acquire a signal function, in which case they facilitated self-regulatory ego functions as defense and compromise were made possible. Intense affect, however, could function to disrupt and overwhelm ego functioning and hence disorganize self-regulation.

Neurobiologists approach this question by detailing the neurochemical mechanisms that mediate affective functions. Psychophysiology is systematically investigating the bidirectional transduction of psychological and physiological processes that underlie mind–body relations. Neurobiology is also elucidating the operations of the brain systems involved in the processing of emotional information, especially the limbic and cortical circuits that mediate affect and its regulation. There is increasing evidence that the orbitofrontal system plays a major role in affect regulation. This system acts as a recovery mechanism that monitors and autoregulates the duration, frequency, and intensity of both positive and negative affects. This makes possible the ability to use affects as signals and the ability to mobilize a self-comforting capacity that can modulate distressing psychobiological states and reestablish positively toned ones. The essential activity of this system is the adaptive switching of internal bodily states in response to changes in the external environment that are appraised to be personally meaningful. Hence, there is evidence that the orbitofrontal cortex functionally mediates the capacity to empathize with the feelings of others (Mega and Cummings, 1994) and to reflect on internal emotional states, one's own and those of others (Povinelli and Preuss, 1995). This orbitofrontal function then mediates "the ability to alter behavior in response to fluctuations in the emotional significance of stimuli" (Dias, Robbins, and Roberts, 1996, p. 69). Schore (1997) maintains that, "in its unique position at the convergence point of right cortical and subcortical systems," the orbitofrontal cortex "critically influences the superior role that the nonverbal right brain plays in the control of vital functions supporting survival and enabling the organism to cope actively and passively with stress and external challenge" (p. 824).

Although approaching affects at the level of brain functioning is vastly different from trying to understand the ways in which they influence psychic functioning, Shore's description of the orbitofrontal cortex is remarkably similar to Freud's explanation of the system ego. It was Freud, first in 1895 in his abandoned "Project" and later in his 1926 treatise on anxiety, who first suggested that affects could function as signals, contributing to self-regulation. He was convinced that brain activity had a crucial role in ego functioning, but at the time he did not have the tools to discover these neurobiological underpinnings. He gave up the Project in frustration and turned toward psychological understanding. Gradually, a comprehensive and increasingly complex psychoanalytic theory of the mind and its functioning evolved. In more recent years, this theory has come to be complemented with greater understanding about the ways in which early experiences influence later psychic functioning.

With greater understanding of the neurobiological substructure that supports Freud's hypothetical self-regulatory system ego, might we have reached a place in which greater collaboration between psychoanalysis and neurobiology is possible, both in the realm of developmental research and intervention? Do we know the developmental trajectory of this orbitofrontal system? Do we understand those factors that lead to the formation of a system that functions optimally or those factors that lead to a system that functions less than adequately? Are there certain behavioral referents that provide clues as to optimal or dysfunctional metabolic activity in the orbitofrontal cortex? In other words, can we translate recent neurobiological breakthroughs into clinically useful tools? Or, might greater integration of the psychodynamic understanding of early childhood behaviors and neurobiological understanding of brain functioning be a necessary first step toward a more complete understanding of the development of an optimally functioning orbitofrontal system? This understanding might serve as a guide for developing clinically useful tools and tools that might provide for more effective early intervention. Early reports of PET imaging studies suggest that with successful psychological treatment patients show significant changes in metabolic activity in the right orbitofrontal cortex and its subcortical connections. Perhaps early childhood intervention would be even more effective than later psychotherapy in facilitating the optimal functioning of this system.

Clearly this would be an exciting but extremely ambitious project, well beyond the scope of this paper. Therefore, I concentrate on the psychoanalytic understanding of the developmental roots of affect regulation so that we might be able to refine our current clinical tools in dealing with adolescents less able to regulate affect.

PSYCHOANALYTIC THEORY OF AFFECT REGULATION

To understand what makes affect regulation possible for one adolescent and not another, we must consider the developmental and functional

26

interaction among affects, object relations, motivation, and self-regulation.

In a way, psychic balance is always temporary, precarious, and unstable. Once established, it is easily jarred and disturbed. Ideally, minor shifts in equilibrium can be regulated without stormy upheavals. That is, the signal function of affect is operating; small samplings of affect are perceived and can be reflected upon. Defenses can be mobilized so that the individual can find whatever compromise is needed to avoid the danger, and balance can be reestablished. Functioning in this way, affects safeguard self-regulation. This signal function is not a given; it must develop alongside other emerging ego functions.

Affects can also disorganize psychic functioning. At times, danger is not forestalled. Whether it be loss of control of an impulse from the inside, or an event experienced, feelings of intense fear, anxiety, anger, sexual excitement, and the like are experienced. The intensity of these feelings may totally overwhelm self-regulatory efforts, in which case feelings of panic or rage are predominant. Such a disruption can be traumatic. Because of the immaturity of the psyche, trauma in early childhood can leave major psychic scars. Repeated traumas over the course of childhood, or growing up in an environment characterized by constant turmoil, little predictability, and affectively misattuned caregivers with few resources to help reestablish equilibrium, can undermine the development of any self-regulatory system. Although psychoanalysts have long observed this phenomenon clinically (Greenacre, 1941; Bergman and Escalona, 1949; Khan, 1963; A. Freud, 1967; Weil, 1970, 1978; Call, 1983), neurobiological studies are beginning to demonstrate a relation between stressful early environments and a less than optimally functioning corticolimbic system (Schore, 1994, 1996, 1997). We now have more definitive data demonstrating that stressful, chaotic, pathological environments undermine self-regulatory development and that, consequently, affects, anxiety in particular, instead of serving a signal function, become readily generated and ingrained in an individual's character structure. Not only is self-regulation easily disrupted, but it is readily generated, and pervasive anxiety leads to chronic disregulation and dysfunctional patterns of relating to others; attempts to manipulate, control, and blame others serve as meager substitutes for self-control.

The infant–caregiver relationship[1] provides the envelope from which the child's psychic functioning emerges. We may then wonder if there

---

[1]Throughout this paper, I refer to the caregiver as the mother, recognizing that this could be mother, father, other, or a composite of all.

is something (and, if so, what it is) in this early mother–child relationship that contributes to a child's (and later to an adolescent's) developing the capacity to use the signal function of affect.

SIGNAL FUNCTION DEVELOPMENT

Spitz (1962, 1963) introduced the idea of mother–infant reciprocity because he wanted to emphasize the importance of a two-way meaningful communication process—an affective dialogue between mother and infant. He thought that this dialogue provided the basis for object relations and for self-regulatory ego functioning. Neurobiological studies now support these suppositions, for there is growing evidence suggesting that representations of affectively meaningful relationships act as "biological regulators" (Schore, 1997).

Fonagy et al. (1993) add that a psychological self (i.e., a sense of self that can see itself and the object world in terms of feelings, beliefs, intentions, and desires—a self that can reflect upon experience in terms of mental states) also emerges through this intersubjective process. Such a capacity further facilitates self-regulation.

Although the baby is born with a primitive physiological capacity for self-regulation, it is the mother who nurtures and supports its homeostasis and regulates social interactions in the beginning. She does this not only by timely response to the infant's signal of hunger and distress, but also by vocal and facial affective expressions. Very gradually, the infant begins to attribute subjective meaning to these expressions; the form and meaning they come to have as well as the ways in which they are transformed and modified will be determined by the valence of the affective interaction.

By 8 months we see a shift, and the baby begins a more active role in self-regulation. She does this by beginning to use the mother's affective expressions. A new toy, a strange person, or a strange situation, and the baby looks to the mother's affective expression; an approving smile, and the baby explores; a fearful or disapproving frown, and the baby bursts into tears. Now mother must help the baby make the transition to a calmer state. This so-called social referencing (Sorce, Emde, and Klinnert, 1981; Emde and Sorce, 1983) continues throughout life; a notable example is when Karen, particularly when she is anxious, such as when she is talking about her sexual feelings, looks to my face for a judgmental frown or a supportive smile.

Usually by about 18 months the infant demonstrates a capacity for representational and symbolic thinking, evident in self-recognition as well as receptive and evocative speech. Now the inner and outer worlds can be ordered, categorized, and labeled, at least in some primitive fashion. With these tools, the child can also begin to develop the capacity for self-reflection (Fonagy et al., 1993). If the mother provides a "good enough" mental mirror (Winnicott, 1967), which in this case also includes labeling mental states (feelings, beliefs, desires, intentions), the child gradually, over time, begins to recognize these in the other and then in the self and to reflect upon them. Recognition and eventual labeling of affects provide the potential for control (Katan, 1961).

Ordering, categorizing, and labeling wishes, directives, and feeling states brings the young child face to face with incompatible aims. He comes to recognize that his feelings and desires and those of his mother are not always identical; he wants his own way, and he wants that comfortable feeling of "fitting together" that only mother in her loving moments can provide.

Faced with conflict—between wishes for gratification and mother's prohibition, between wishes for gratification and wishes for mother's love—the young child may begin to experience intense angry feelings. When power and control come to be prevalent themes in the relationship, as they often do, anger can intensify. Yet, feeling intensely angry may lead the young child to feel a loss of the loving connection with mother. Anger is easily projected, and, instead of an object of safety, mother may be seen as a feared punishing figure. The young child can then feel desperately helpless and overwhelmed with anxiety, particularly as symbolic thinking provides the capacity for the lurid fantasy elaboration of possible consequences we know to be characteristic of young children. Great demands are now made upon immature self-regulatory functions.

Great demands are also now placed on the mother. She is called upon to be consistent, to maintain her perspective, to respond to the child's affective signals with regulatory, safety-keeping interventions, and to help the young child find adaptive ways of expressing anger and other unpleasant emotions. Ideally, the mother's response to affective signals is timely and effective before affects escalate. If she can avoid becoming overly distressed by the young child's anger, demands, or distress and avoid being drawn into the struggle, she can respond to emotional storms with a regulating balance. That is, she may tolerate some drive expression, yet she expects certain compliance and so facilitates compromise. This ensures that the toddler's affective storms do not reach proportions that undermine self-regulation. And yet, appropriate experiences of delay encourage the building of frustration tolerance and self-coping skills and offer the child the opportunity to feel a sense of pride in successful mastery.

If the mother is successful in her role as what some call an "auxiliary ego" and others call a selfobject, identification with her as part of the process of separation and individuation will include identification with her many functions—demands for drive restraint, soothing functions, identification with her recognition and timely regulatory response to affective signals, and identification with her capacity to find compromise. The child becomes decreasingly vulnerable to feeling overwhelmed and disorganized by affects, for they can be identified as they arise, before they reach overwhelming proportions. The child can then take appropriate self-defensive measures, and self-regulatory and self-organizational capacities mature alongside developing object relations.

Loewald (1979), in discussing optimal resolution of early childhood conflict, particularly the complicated and conflictual wishes associated with the Oedipus complex, maintained that more than guilt, self-punishment, and repression were necessary to cope with oedipal conflict. What was also needed was mastery, assuming self-responsibility, or "owning up to one's needs and impulses as one's own." This means coming to terms with the differences in sexes and in generations, with what one is and is not entitled to, with the fact that not only do parents make rules but that they also must live by a conventional set of rules. Instead of having feelings of guilt and self-punishment after the fact, an individual must come to a stabilized code of internal rules and ethics and learn to live within those internalized rules. Such self-responsibility is achieved only gradually, over developmental time. However, the extent to which the child can engage in the more complex object relations we associate with oedipal fantasies and wishes and adaptively master the conflicts of the associated sexual and aggressive impulses may depend on the extent to which the child can efficiently use the signal function of affect to ensure self-regulation.

Early childhood fantasies, wishes, and conflicts underlie adolescent interpersonal relationships with parents, teachers, peers, and lovers. As in early childhood, an adolescent's success in adaptively mastering adolescent conflicts and his ability and willingness to take responsibility for actions and motivations will also depend on the degree to which the adolescent can efficiently use the signal function of affect to ensure self-regulation.

Psychopathology

With this framework of normal development as a backdrop, we turn to the challenge of understanding the adolescent patient who fails to regulate affect. We have to keep in mind several factors and the ways in which they are interdependent. First, patterns of interacting form early, and they endure. Early patterns are reflected in the ways in which our patients relate to us, their parents, and their peers, and these patterns will influence the ways in which parents eventually relate to their children, as the patterns are passed from one generation to the next. Object relations influence the development of psychic systems, the do's and don'ts of inner rules and morals, as well as the organizing, self-regulatory ego functions. Psychopathology in the early mother–child relationship that results in deficient self-regulatory skills renders an adolescent less able to manage anxiety-prone situations.

Greta is an example. Needless to say, she refused treatment at the time I saw her. Instead, she became pregnant and secretly married her boyfriend. By the time the baby was born, she was hopelessly addicted to crack and alcohol. Her mother was appointed legal guardian of her baby while she spent the next 18 months in and out of drug treatment facilities. Interestingly, I learned that her actions reflected those of her mother, who also had become pregnant at an early age, had run away from home, and had had several husbands subsequent to Greta's father. Neither Greta nor her mother had adequate problem-solving skills. With little capacity for self-observation and self-regulation, neither could take responsibility for her actions, each blamed others for her plight, and each looked to others to provide solutions to her problems.

In optimal development of a capacity for affective regulation, I mentioned first the importance of the attuned mother's entering into an affective dialogue with her infant, thereby maintaining a sense of safety. At times the mother fails, and the infant's tensions escalate. This may be because of the temperament of the infant, neurological immaturity or defect, or because mother herself is emotionally unavailable, overanxious, unpredictable, unstable, or overwhelmed. The infant may then experience persistent, diffuse tension states and archaic excitations. These may lead to exaggerated and skewed drive expressions as well as predispose the infant to a state of anxiety readiness, all of which is recorded in neuronal patterning. Later, the effects of genetic defect and early environmental stress are impossible to distinguish neurologically. Not able to experience the mother's loving investment, the distressed, difficult-to-calm infant is unable to return signals that reinforce the mother's confidence in her mothering skills. Instead of a synchronized loving bond, attachment may be disturbed, and the anxiety-prone infant may become the recipient of projection—perceived as a "monster" bent on persecuting mother. As one mother, describing her four-month old daughter, exclaimed, "She's just angry, mean, manipulating. But what should I expect? The first time I saw her, she gave me a cold, icy stare and looked away."

A constant, relatively high level of anxiety readiness precedes and intensifies ordinary expectable phase-specific developmental conflicts. The amorphous tension of a dysfunctional household, which is often highly charged with uncontrolled sexuality and aggression, may lead the child to libidinize distress and anxiety. The child may then experience a suffusion of the entire organism with sexual excitations involving premature and excessive genital stimulation or a high level of aggressive potential. There tends to be a primitive interconnection between anxiety and rage. So frequently, the forceful self-expression coming from a toddler limited in skill and repertoire for self-expression is mistaken as anger. The response of the environment usually determines what happens next. A mother's supportive response can further the development of adaptive self-assertion; an angry, punitive, or attacking response leads to anxiety, dysregulation, and then rage. The so-called temper tantrum of a toddler is usually more an indication of anxiety and disorganization rather than an expression of rage. Repetitive stressful situations excessively challenge the young child's task of learning to tolerate ambivalence and come to terms with libidinal and aggressive impulses. Anger provides a special challenge to the toddler in the throes of rapprochement ambivalence. This anger is easily projected, which, in combination with the lurid fantasies, sexual excitation, and fears typical of very young children, leads the child to anticipate abandonment, loss of love, castration, or other bodily damage. These expectations then lead a child to experience even a "good enough" mother as bad. The feared maternal imago lends credence to fears of loss of love and/or to fears of castration, and such fears further undermine object relations and self-regulation.

In early childhood, the child "uses" the mother to calm his anxiety and regulate his emotional storms. Ideally, the young child uses his mother to learn adaptive ways of handling intense emotions and uses her to learn to use affects as a warning signal so as to avoid overwhelming distress. Winnicott (1969) observes, however, that at times, particularly in early childhood, little differentiation is made between object and subject, and perception of the mother is colored by the child's own impulses, affects, and projections. Winnicott stresses that, if the object is to be used, "it must be real in the sense of being part of shared reality, not a bundle of projections" (p. 88). That is, the mother must behave differently from the child's projection-based expectations. He must experience that she does not feel threatened and frightened by his emotions and is not stimulated or manipulated to respond in kind to him. Instead, she must feel and be able to convey that a sense of continuing safety prevails despite the child's affective storm. For example, in response to a mother's restriction, the child may have murderous fantasies and erupt in rage. Mother's role is to be in charge. She must reassure the child that his angry, murderous thoughts do not frighten, hurt, or kill her, nor do they provoke her to attack in response. If she can tolerate the child's affects, not be manipulated to give in or retaliate, and intervene in a timely way, he can gradually begin to distinguish between his own inner world and the reality of the mother. He can then "use" the mother's regulating, safety-keeping functions to quiet his emotional storms and calm his anxiety and "use" his mother to learn adaptive ways of managing his angry feelings. It is in this way that the capacity to use affects as signals to organize ego functioning effectively depends on successful use of and identification with the mother.

It is in this most basic area that the relationship between child and parent often breaks down. That is, not only is there lacking a clear differentiation between child and parent in the child's mind, but often in the parent's mind as well. Sometimes a crying baby is viewed as crying deliberately to interrupt mother's sleep; the toddler is seen to be willfully and purposefully getting into everything to make a mess for mother; and the angry toddler is viewed as an uncontrollable monster. Because such a mother is herself unable to use affective signals, she fails miserably in mastering the adaptive use of aggression. Therefore, she is easily drawn into and provoked by the toddler's challenges, and, identifying with the child's projections, she erupts in rage and attacks her young child. Or, she avoids confrontation for fear that her anger (as well as her child's) is uncontrollable. A mother of a three-year-old explained to me that she was unable to take her child to a toy store for fear he would want everything in the store. She described that, during the last visit, he had a huge temper tantrum when he was refused a toy. This mother admitted to having nightmares of killing her child when he was a baby. Her terror of losing control of her repressed angry impulses rendered her incapable of assertively and constructively setting firm limits. Instead, to avoid public humiliation as well as to assure herself that her child loved her, she gave in. At times, however, she admitted that she became enraged by his behavior and was forced to isolate herself for fear of losing control, functionally abandoning her child when she was needed most.

Frequently mothers failure to recognize that the boundary between themselves and their child extends to the child's body. When angry, such parents feel entitled to invade and physically abuse the child's body. One particularly articulate four-year-old described her utter confusion. Her mother spanked her with a hairbrush. Why? She hit her sister. Why was mother entitled to hit her, but she was not permitted to communicate in the same way? Clearly, the mother's using physical abuse as a means of resolving conflict taught the daughter that conflict is best resolved with physical force. Should we be surprised that adolescents with such early histories do not hesitate to use physical attack on others as a response to frustration and as a means of resolving conflict?

Another mother responded to my suggestion of holding to firm limits to avoid affective escalations by saying that such an idea made her feel mean. She recognized that she often feels mean when her child challenges her directives, and so she frequently gives in. However, she admitted that at times she feels enraged and loses control when her daughter does not pay any attention to her when she does set limits. She failed to see the connection. Interestingly, Greta's mother was at a loss to understand Greta's unhappy rebellion. She had tried to be a good mother, not to set rules, restrictions. Greta could do just about anything she wanted. This approach had failed to give Greta a sense of safety, a tolerance for frustration, and problem-solving tools. Instead, both Greta and her mother felt unloved and unsafe. Such a mother cannot be "used," in Winnicott's sense. Instead, varieties of sadomasochistic, manipulative, or other maladaptive behaviors substitute for effective dialogue.

The object-related conflicts of early childhood become internalized and form the matrix for a developing inner system of prohibitions and restraints. When young children are not able to "use" their parents in the manner I have described, such development is delayed and impaired. Early childhood wishes and conflicts are not mastered by internalization and identification with the rules of parents and society, and so no responsibility is taken for their wishes and actions. As adolescents, such individuals frequently become preoccupied with narcissistic issues related to omnipotent demands for control and/or domination. They easily erupt in rage when they cannot control the outside world. They blame others for their problems and feel cheated and victimized. Feeling cheated allows them to feel justified in not living up to the rules of their family or society, as they feel entitled to get now what they think they missed. They take little responsibility for their actions and feel dependent on others to make them feel better. The responsibility for change is therefore relegated to the external world. For these individuals, instead of a consistently loving inner presence and the capacity to self-regulate, they appear to have a consistently negative relationship with a critical, easily projected inner object (Blum, 1981). The persistent tendency to split object representations into idealized and devalued, good and bad, persecutory and protective, makes affect regulation and self-responsibility extremely difficult. An adolescent with such a clinical picture suggests a failure in learning to tolerate ambivalence and to find some balance between the libidinal and aggressive forces within their personalities. These adolescents may have a capacity for attachment, as they cling tenaciously to abusive boyfriends or repeat abusive patterns of relating with girlfriends, but they have not formed a capacity to use affects as signals to ensure self-regulation.

Karen's boyfriend is an example. He seemed to have only tenuous control over anxiety and saw any slight, any criticism, any rejection (e.g., frustration of his sexual overtures and desires) as a threat to his masculinity, as a castration threat. Any slight disagreement with Karen, and he became enraged and verbally and physically abusive. He seemed to feel little remorse or guilt and instead displaced this onto Karen (as she later came to find out) as he saw her and most women as inferior, dependent, childish, frivolous; they were the ones who were sexually seductive, taking advantage of him. Any guilt or self-loathing for his angry outbursts or his lack of will to abstain from sexual passions (she found out he also had had several affairs while dating her) became a loathing of the girl, as he justified his behavior. He clearly did not seem to feel he had to take responsibility for his own actions, for he saw Karen as responsible.

Karen's own unresolved conflicts of early childhood were revived in her adolescent struggles with her boyfriend and her mother. Unresolved ambivalence toward the mother as well as guilt for oedipal sexual fantasies often leads a young girl to fear her mother's destructive envy of any attention she may have from her father. Derivatives of this conflict may lead an adolescent girl to feel guilty about any sexual desires she may have toward a man. Fantasies of being raped are frequently defensive solutions to such conflicts for adolescent girls. In such fantasies, the girl's own sexual desire is disavowed and disguised as she makes herself the victim of another's desire. The sexuality is further disguised by the aggressive manifest content. Such fantasies, coupled with dependency needs, often lead a girl into self-destructive, unsafe situations and abusive relationships. She then may cling to the abusive partner, fearing that being alone would be far worse than being abused. Such was the story of Karen, and she felt devastated and hopeless when he finally left her. Although Prozac helped lift her depression, it did not remove the pain or help her to discover her vulnerability to such relationships.

Conclusion

As we race toward the millennium, we are striving mightily to keep up with the technological advances that make brain study possible. We are also scrambling to keep abreast with the advances in knowledge these studies bring and to extend studies further. Technology has also brought increasingly effective ways of psychopharmacological management of affective disorders. Yet, adolescents continue to cry out for help with their psychological distress. Perhaps it would behoove us to stop and take note of the implications of our fast moving society. What does it mean that fewer and fewer children are growing up in intact families; that more and more children are being raised in day-care and after-school-care situations; that children are exposed to increasingly violent themes through the media and their ever so popular video games; and that the majority of parent–child interactions take place during times of stress—when everybody is trying to get out of the house in the morning, or when mother is exhausted after a long day's work and is trying to prepare dinner and everybody is cranky and hungry? Do our current life styles produce more and more children less skilled in affect regulation? Can our psychopharmacological tools meet the needs of the child who has not learned to use affects as early warning signs? Can psychopharmacological intervention correct a skewed developmental trajectory of the orbitofrontal cortex? Can managed care support the kinds of intervention that may be needed later?

I have attempted to make a small contribution, from a psychoanalytic perspective, of one possible developmental factor that may make affect regulation in adolescence particularly challenging. Acknowledging that genetic and neurobiological determinants contribute, I have suggested that the capacity to use the signal function of affects to maintain self-regulation may largely determine whether an adolescent will be able to adaptively manage the inner flux and change brought by the biological changes of adolescence or else be overwhelmed by the *Sturm und Drang*. Although the signal function of affect may be understood by neurobiology as the role of the orbitofrontal system, we might also be able to predict the later metabolic functioning of this system by paying attention to the early mother–child relationship. In understanding the way in which optimal functioning of the signal function is rooted in early mother–child interactions, we might be better equipped to understand our therapeutic interactions with our adolescent patients. If we can avoid identification with their projections and tolerate and eventually help them contain their emotional storms, perhaps they might be better able to trust us and to "use" us to answer to their cry.

REFERENCES

Bergman, P. & Escalona, S. K. (1949), Unusual sensitivities in very young children. *The Psychoanalytic Study of the Child,* 3:333–352. New York: International Universities Press.

Blos, P. (1967), The second individuation process of adolescence. *The Psychoanalytic Study of the Child,* 22:162–186. New York: International Universities Press.

Blum, H. (1981), Object inconstancy and paranoid conspiracy. *J. Amer. Psychoanal. Assn.,* 29:789–814.

Call, J. (1983), Toward a nosology of psychiatric disorders in infancy. In: *Frontiers of Infant Psychiatry,* ed. J. D. Call, E. Galenson & R. L. Tyson. New York: Basic Books, pp. 117–128.

Dias, R., Robbins, T. W. & Roberts, A. C. (1996), Dissociation in prefrontal cortex of affective and attentional shifts. *Nature*, 380:69–72.

Emde, R. N. & Sorce, J. F. (1983), The rewards of infancy: Emotional availability and maternal referencing. In: *Frontiers of Infant Psychiatry*, ed. J. D. Call, E. Galenson & R. L. Tyson. New York: Basic Books, pp. 17–30.

Feinstein, S. C., Giovacchini, P. & Miller, A., ed. (1971), *Adolescent Psychiatry: Vol 1. Developmental and Clinical Studies*. New York: Basic Books.

Fonagy, P., Moran, G. S., Edgecumbe, R., Kennedy, H. & Target, M. (1993), The roles of mental representations and processes in therapeutic action. *The Psychoanalytic Study of the Child*, 48:9–48. New York: International Universities Press.

Freud, A. (1967), Comments on psychic trauma. In: *The Writings of Anna Freud: Vol. 5*. New York: International Universities Press, 1969, pp. 221–241.

Freud, S. (1926), Inhibitions, symptoms and anxiety. *Standard Edition*, 20:77–175. London: Hogarth Press, 1959.

Greenacre, P. (1941), The predisposition to anxiety. In: *Trauma, Growth and Personality*. New York: Norton, 1952, pp. 27–82.

Katan, A. (1961), Some thoughts about the role of verbalization in early childhood. *The Psychoanalytic Study of the Child*, 16:184–188. New York: International Universities Press.

Khan, M. M. R. (1963), The concept of cumulative trauma. *The Psychoanalytic Study of the Child*, 18:286–306. New York: International Universities Press.

Loewald, H. (1979), The waning of the Oedipus complex. In: *Papers on Psychoanalysis*. New Haven, CT: Yale University Press, 1980, 384–404.

Mahler, M. S., Pine, F. & Bergman, A. (1975), *The Psychological Birth of the Human Infant*. New York: Basic Books.

Mega, M. S. & Cummings, J. L. (1994), Frontal-subcortical circuits and neuropsychiatric disorders. *J. of Neuropsychiatry & Clinical Neuroscience*, 6:358–370.

Povinelli, D. & Preuss, T. M. (1995), Theory of mind: Evolutionary history of a cognitive specialization. *Trends in Neuroscience*, 18:418–424.

Schore, A. (1994), *Affect Regulation and Origin of the Self*. Hillsdale, NJ: Lawrence Erlbaum Associates.

——— (1996), The experience-dependent maturation of a regulatory system in the orbital prefrontal cortex and the origin of developmental psychopathology. *Develop. & Psychopathol.*, 8:59–87.

——— (1997), A century after Freud's project: Is rapprochement between psychoanalysis and neurobiology at hand? *J. Amer. Psychoanal. Assn.*, 45:807–840.

Sorce, J. F., Emde, R. N. & Klinnert, M. (1981), Maternal emotional signaling: Its effect on the visual-cliff behavior of one-year-olds. Presented at meeting of the Society for Research in Child Development, Boston.

Spitz, R. (1962), Autoerotism re-examined: Early sexual behavior and personality. *The Psychoanalytic Study of the Child*, 17:238–318. New York: International Universities Press.

——— (1963), Life and the dialogue. In: *Counterpoint: Libidinal Object and Subject*, ed. H. S. Gaskill. New York: International Universities Press, pp. 154–176.

Weil, A. (1970), The basic core. *The Psychoanalytic Study of the Child*, 25:442–460. New York: International Universities Press.

——— (1978), Maturational variations and genetic-dynamic issues. *J. Amer. Psychoanal. Assn.*, 26:461–492.

Winnicott, D. W. (1967), Mirror-role of mother and family in child development. In: *Playing with Reality*. New York: Basic Books.

——— (1969), The use of an object. *Internat. J. Psycho-Anal.*, 50:711–716.

3 THE ROLE OF FAMILY INTERACTIONS IN ADOLESCENT DEPRESSION: A REVIEW OF RESEARCH FINDINGS

STEVEN H. KATZ

It may seem obvious that parents are a very important influence in an adolescent's life and that adolescents are sensitive to and affected by their parents' behaviors. However, research that tests these beliefs in cases of adolescent depression has only recently blossomed. This relative neglect by researchers is understandable. Until the early 1980s, most theorists believed that young people are not capable of being clinically depressed (Rie, 1966; Cantwell and Carlson, 1983). There has also been considerable difficulty in measuring something as fluid as family interactions (Jacobs, 1975). Luckily, there have recently been important theoretical advances. These include the understanding that young people do have depressive episodes and that parental depression is a risk factor for adolescent depression because parenting skills get eroded. There have been diagnostic advances as well. These include clear diagnostic criteria similar to those for adults. Finally, there have been methodological advances. These include the development of reliable observational coding systems, the use of videotaped interactions, and better research on self-report measures. All of these advances have improved our ability to make more definite statements about common interaction patterns in families with a depressed adolescent.

Researchers have found that there are many factors that contribute to adolescent depression. These factors include the child's temperament, the parents' child-rearing practices, the parents' marital distress, family

An earlier version of this chapter was presented at the meeting of the International Society for Adolescent Psychiatry, Chicago, June 13, 1992.

economic status, stressful life events, biochemical and genetic factors, depressive cognitions, and peer and school factors. But, most of these factors exert their influence through family interactions. Although peers may become an equally or more important socializing agent when a child reaches adolescence, family interaction still has an impact and remains an important place to intervene when an adolescent becomes depressed.

Depression in adolescence represents a persistent disruption of normal development and of self-esteem functioning. Although only 5% or fewer of adolescents are clinically depressed, about 20% report significant depressive symptoms (Kashani, Carlson, and Beck, 1987). Adolescent depression can be lengthy and recurrent. It represents a risk factor for continued psychopathology and poorer psychosocial adjustment as an adult. It is often accompanied by other disorders, most notably conduct disorders, anxiety, and substance abuse (Kovacs et al., 1984a, b; Marriage et al., 1986).

This chapter reviews studies that have asked, "Are there family interaction patterns, behaviors, or characteristics that are regularly found in families with a depressed adolescent?" Researchers have gone about answering this question in three ways. First, they have had adolescents complete self-report measures about their family environments or have had depressed adults report about their youth. Second, they have examined families with a depressed mother. Third, they have measured family interactions in depressed youth directly through observations.

The research presented in this review generally uses samples of subjects who self-reported symptoms of depression or met diagnostic criteria for major depression or dysthymia as described in the *Diagnostic and Statistical Manual of Mental Disorders, 3rd Edition–Revised* (American Psychiatric Association, 1987). Although this chapter focuses on depressed adolescents, results from studies with younger children and with depressed adults and from studies that used less stringent diagnostic criteria are included when they add insight into family patterns.

Self-Report Studies of Family Environments

Self-report studies have tested the hypotheses that, compared with families of nondepressed people, families of depressed people are more rejecting, less cohesive, or more overprotecting. Also, the hypothesis has been tested that the depressed person's view of the family's functioning is divergent from the view of the rest of his family. Third, self-report studies have examined a variety of structural variables such as family intactness and marital conflict. Each of these dimensions is examined in turn.

REJECTION

Research findings have consistently found that depressed children, adolescents, and adults, as well as parents of depressed youth, report or recall greater parental rejection and hostility than nondepressed subjects (Puig-Antich et al., 1985a, b; Koestner, Zuroff, and Powers, 1991). A good example of this research is the Koestner, Zuroff, and Powers (1991) study of 12-year-olds whose mothers had earlier completed a research protocol when their children were 5. They found that mother-reported parenting behaviors of restrictiveness and rejection when her child was 5 years old were correlated with the child's being self-critical at age 12. This relation held while controlling for mother's report of the child's temperament before age 5. This finding suggests that rejection of the child may lead to the children's reinforcing themselves in the same strict and nonaccepting manner that their parents demanded of them. A critique of the studies focused on rejection, however, is that most of them used currently depressed subjects. This design feature is significant, as some researchers find that the perception of parents as rejecting is a function of the subject being currently depressed (Lewinsohn and Rosenbaum, 1987), although other studies found that perceptions of negative parenting were stable at least 3 years beyond the depressive episode (Gotlib et al., 1988).

COHESION, ADAPTABILITY, AND OVERPROTECTION

Several self-report studies have used measures of family cohesion and adaptability. Cohesion is the emotional bonding that family members have toward one another. This variable ranges from enmeshment (an overidentification with the family) to disengagement (characterized by low bonding and high autonomy). Adaptability is the flexibility (from rigidity to chaos) of the family in response to stress (Olson, Bell, and Portner, 1982).

Most studies found that low cohesion was significantly correlated with depression scores. For example, Fendrich, Warner, and Weissman (1990) found that children and adolescents who reported low cohesion in their family had a four-fold increased risk for depression than subjects who did not report it. Research has also suggested that depressed adolescents and adults report their parents to be "guilt inducing" rather than punishing and to be overprotective, emotionally distant, and rigid in their child-rearing attitudes and practices (Brook et al., 1983; Susman et al., 1985; Hetherington and Martin, 1986; Gotlib et al., 1988). Thus, the perception that one's parents are unavailable, inflexible, or overprotective appears to be correlated with, and possibly results in, the experience of depression.

CONGRUENCE BETWEEN FAMILY MEMBERS' PERCEPTIONS

Another risk factor that emerges from the literature is that depressed (especially suicidal depressed) individuals hold a view of themselves or some major aspect of their family's functioning that is markedly at odds with the views of other family members. This pattern has been found in comparing depressed inpatients with other family members (Keitner et al., 1987; Miller et al., 1986), adolescents with low self-esteem with their parents (Offer, Ostrov, and Howard, 1982), depressed college students with their siblings (Oliver et al., 1987; Lopez, Campbell, and Watkins, 1989), and depressed children with their parents (Stark et al., 1990).

These family studies suggest that depressed adolescents, more so than nondepressed individuals, may hold perceptions of their family environments that are not shared by other family members. This discrepancy may be a consequence of, or a contributing factor to, the depression. Either way, if the family's perceptions are sufficiently different from the adolescent's, it becomes less likely that the adolescent will be able to make use of the family as a helping resource. For example, when an adolescent, relative to other family members, perceives the family to be less affectively expressive, to observe poorer role boundaries, or to have poorer control over behavior, then negative consequences may ensue for this adolescent. The adolescent may then not find the family to be much of a resource in helping him or her cope with stress, feelings of isolation may increase, and it may feel impossible to communicate in the "family's language" about troubling problems and feelings.

FAMILY INTACTNESS AND MARITAL CONFLICT

Several studies suggest that parental loss, divorce or single-parenting, and high marital conflict can all result in child depression. Early studies of depression in youth focused on the trauma resulting from losing or being separated from a parent. The results indicated that parental loss during childhood or adolescence increases the risk of depression in adulthood by a factor of two to three times. Losing either parent during the period of birth to 5 years and father loss from 10 to 14 years were especially traumatic (Birtchnell, 1970; Barnes and Prosen, 1985). But, given that only a small portion of depressed youth experienced loss of a parent, other factors must be operative. More recent studies have found that such factors as the quality of pre-loss marriage (Harris and Howard, 1987), high maternal indifference before the loss (Bifulco, Brown, and Harris, 1987), and parental care after the loss (Klerman et al., 1984; Breier et al., 1988) mediate the relationship between parent loss and child depression.

Some studies have found more self-reported depression in the children of divorced or single parents. Only Asarnow, Carlson, and Perdue (1988), however, utilized clinician-diagnosed depressed children and adolescents. They found, interestingly, that more children in their sample with major depression came from two-parent families than children with dysthymic disorder (73% vs. 56%). However, as was true for the parent-loss studies, more recent studies have gone further to show that other variables mediate this relationship. These studies indicate that family process variables account for the association between family intactness and depression rather than divorce or single-parenting per se. These variables include degree of parent involvement, parent–adolescent conflict, marital conflict, and communication problems (Emery, 1982; Shaw and Emery, 1987; Feldman, Rubenstein, and Rubin, 1988; Tesser et al., 1989).

With regard to marital conflict, studies have been mixed as to whether there is more marital conflict in families with a depressed adolescent (Emery, 1982; Puig-Antich et al., 1985b). As might be expected, studies that measured both marital conflict and parent–adolescent conflict found the latter to be more predictive of child internalizing problems (Forehand et al., 1988).

Depressed Parents

Studies of depressed mothers and their children are important because as many as 40% to 50% of the children of a depressed parent have a diagnosable psychiatric disturbance. These children have approximately three times the rate of affective disorder and six times the rate of major depressive disorder (Cytryn et al., 1982; Orvashel, Welsh-Allis, and Weijai, 1988; Downey and Coyne, 1990). Although some researchers have not found that normal parents demonstrate better parenting than depressed parents (Goodman and Brumley, 1990), most studies do find group differences.

Although genetic factors are often cited as causes here, psychosocial factors are also clearly implicated. Studies have found that the older the children, the less likely they are to be adversely affected by maternal depression (Burbach and Borduin, 1986; Weissman et al., 1987). For example, Weissman et al. (1987) found that, in a group of depressed children and teens, those that had one or both depressed parents became depressed at a younger age than if neither parent was depressed (12.7 vs. 16.8 years). One way to understand these findings is that a depressed parent's disturbed psychosocial processes are in part responsible for the transmission of depression. Adolescents with their stronger sense of self would presumably be less vulnerable to these disturbing interactions than young children. Also, Hammen, Burge, and Adrian (1991) demonstrated that, in a sample of depressed children and adolescents, the onset of their symptoms was temporally associated with the occurrence of symptoms in their mothers. In other words, the children's depressive episodes predictably followed their mothers' episodes. Hammen et al. conceptualized the mechanism at work as an absence of supportive parenting by the depressed mother—parenting that might buffer stress in the children's lives. These parenting deficits eventually translate into poorer child functioning.

DEPRESSED MOTHERS AND THEIR INFANTS

To understand more specifically how depression in a parent affects the child, it is useful to look at the field of infant research. The field of infant research is notable for developing reliable coding systems used to rate observed mother–child interactions. Studies of infants in interaction have found that depressed mothers typically exhibit flat affect and provide less stimulation and less responsiveness toward their infants or young children. Their infants then show fewer contented expressions, more fussiness, lower activity levels, and poorer attentiveness toward their mothers than do infants of nondepressed mothers (Field, 1984; Field et al., 1985; Cohn et al., 1986). The infants then exhibit these behaviors in their interactions with nondepressed adults (Field et al., 1988).

Studies with children and adolescents have found that depressed parents display less affection and happy affect, have more problems in communicating, show more dysphoric affect, and demonstrate greater ambivalence toward the family than do nondepressed parents (Weissman et al., 1984; Hops et al., 1987). Depressed parents are more critical, power-assertive, and hostile toward their children than nondepressed parents. Dysphoric mothers also suppressed their children's aggressive and command-giving behavior (Friedman, 1984; Biglan et al., 1985; Biglan, Hops, and Sherman, 1988; Hops et al., 1987), and depressed fathers interacting with their sons showed less smiling, laughing, and humor than alcoholic or normal fathers interacting with their sons (Jacobs, Krahn, and Leonard, 1991). Families with a depressed parent are also characterized by less cohesion and expressiveness, more conflict, less emphasis on the development of independence, and fewer shared fun activities (Billings and Moos, 1983). It is notable that the impact of disturbed parenting is reduced when one of the parents does not exhibit these behaviors (Hops et al., 1987; Jacobs et al., 1991).

DEPRESSION AFFECTS PERCEPTION

Depression also appears to affect mothers' perceptions of their children, so that mothers who are depressed see even the normal behavior of their children as depressed (Griest, Wells, and Forehand, 1979; Rogers and Forehand, 1983; Breslau, Davis, and Prabucki, 1988; Dumas, Gibson, and Albin, 1989). However, findings in this area are mixed, as other studies report both that these parents often do not recognize their own children's depression (Cytryn and McKnew, 1980; Kashani et al., 1985) or that they are more accurate observers of their children's problems than even normal mothers (Conrad and Hammen,

1989). In fact, there is a growing literature supporting the hypothesis that depressed subjects are more "realistic" and have less "optimistic illusions" than nondepressed subjects (see Alloy et al., 1990, for a review).

Observational Studies

Direct-observation studies represent a more valid sampling of actual parental practices than retrospective or self-report accounts. Studies of interaction sequences can provide us clues as to behaviors and sequences of behaviors that lead to or maintain the affective disorder (Hass, Clarkin, and Glick, 1985). Observational studies of interactions in families with a clinically depressed adolescent—which include *DSM–III*–type diagnoses, psychiatric control groups, and reliable coding schemes—are both few and recent (Cole and Rehm, 1986; Asarnow, Goldstein, and Ben-Meir, 1988; Forehand et al., 1988; Cook et al., 1990; Tompson et al., 1990; Dadds et al., 1992; Sanders et al., 1992; Donenberg, Nelson, and Weisz, 1993).

The observational studies published so far have measured rates of positive reinforcement, levels of expressed hostility, and communication problems in families with a depressed child or adolescent. In an exemplary study, Cole and Rehm (1986) compared normal control families with either a depressed or nondepressed child seeking treatment in an outpatient clinic. The families were observed interacting as the child played a game that involved rolling a ball through a maze. Mothers of depressed children rewarded their depressed children at much lower rates than either of the other groups, and, when these mothers did congratulate or support their children's performance, it was only after very high levels of achievement. Their children mirrored this in setting higher standards for themselves before stating they had done well.

Three observational studies included a psychiatric control group (Dadds et al., 1992; Sanders et al., 1992; Donenberg et al., 1993). These researchers found that depressed and mixed depressed/conduct-disordered children and adolescents showed depressed affect or submissiveness toward their parents and low levels of conflict and anger. The mixed group looked much like the depressed group of children but was not as deferential. Conduct-disordered–only adolescents showed both depressed and angry affect toward their parents. Parents of mixed depressed/conduct-disordered adolescents were less critical and more positive toward their children than parents of conduct-disordered–only adolescents. These results suggest observable interaction patterns specific to families with a depressed adolescent.

EXPRESSED EMOTION

In the studies of hostility, researchers sequentially coded interactions in the families of disturbed adolescents who have parents with high or low expressed emotion (EE). As Hooley (1990) defines it, "EE reflects the extent to which a patient's closest relative(s) talks about him or her in a critical or hostile way (in talking with an interviewer)" (p. 58). Thus, EE is a negative attitude toward the patient and is not typically used in observational measures of actual communication within families. Researchers who used this construct found it can predict relapse in depressed patients (Hooley, 1990).

For example, Vaughn and Leff (1976) and Hooley, Orley, and Teasdale (1986) correlated relatives' levels of expressed emotion toward schizophrenic and depressed adolescent and adult inpatients with relapse over the next nine months. When the researchers interviewed the patients' relatives, the relatives of schizophrenics and depressives made equal numbers of critical comments. But, for schizophrenics, if a relative made seven or more critical comments to the interviewer, this predicted that the patient would relapse within nine months; for depressed subjects, only two or more critical (or high-EE) comments were predictive of relapse. In fact, the family member's EE, even more than the severity of depression, was the best predictor of depressed patients' relapses.

However, when you divide these relatives into high and low EE based on interviews with a researcher, and then observe them interacting with their disturbed adolescent, the findings are not clear. Results have been mixed as to whether high-EE parents are actually more expressive of hostility in interactions. Thus, relatives who express hostility toward the disturbed adolescent do not appear to do so consistently in interactions (Valone et al., 1984; Cook et al., 1989). Unfortunately, no study has coded interactions between depressed-only adolescents and their high- or low-EE parents.

COMMUNICATION PROBLEMS

A final focus of observational studies with depressed adolescents has been communication problems. Asarnow, Goldstein, and Ben-Meir

(1988) studied depressed and schizophrenic-spectrum disordered (SSD) children and adolescents interacting with their parents. They found that more than half of the depressed youths had at least one parent who demonstrated communication deviance. Communication deviance measures vague, unfocused, and distorted verbal communication patterns. These parent groups differed, however, in that mothers of SSD children were more likely than mothers of depressed children to reciprocate child negativity, whereas mothers of depressed children were more likely than mothers of SSD children to reciprocate child positiveness. In other studies that used self-report measures of family communication, families with a depressed member reported poorer communication than families with an alcoholic, schizophrenic, adjustment-disordered, or bipolar member (Miller et al., 1986).

Another type of communication problem occurs when parents send conflicting messages to their children. These mixed messages include, for example, a positive verbal content but a negative facial expression or tone of voice. Bugental, Kaswan, and Love (1970, 1971, 1972) found that a significantly higher proportion of mothers of disturbed children produced conflicting messages than did the mothers of normal controls (59% vs. 10%). The researchers found that conflicting affective messages predicted aggressiveness but not withdrawal in the children and that children resolve all conflicting messages by accepting the negative component and discounting any positive component.

Conclusions

This review has highlighted and critiqued important ways in which families may contribute to or maintain depression in adolescents. These trends in the research findings give us suggestions for future studies, but, more important, they point out which aspects of the parent–adolescent relationship should be a focus for treatment. Although not all families with a depressed adolescent meet this profile, the following characteristics have found research support. Research suggests that families with a depressed child or adolescent (compared to normal families) tend to show more rejection, more dysphoria, and possibly more overprotectiveness. They are less involved, display less happy affect, are poorer problem-solvers, give less positive-reinforcement, and have poorer role-functioning. Also, the depressed adolescent may have a perception of how the family is functioning that is at odds with those of the rest of the family. Family patterns that received less research support but that deserve further study include the family's use of unfocused or complex communications and being very expressive of hostility.

In addition to identifying these specific family interaction patterns as risk factors for adolescent depression, this review of research on the role of family relations in child and adolescent depression suggests six important conclusions:

1. Chronic or entrenched family interaction patterns, more so than any individual pathogenic events or traumas, are most likely responsible for depression in children and adolescents.
2. Research has not conclusively demonstrated that these patterns predict depression specifically and not psychopathology in general.
3. Research converges in suggesting that it is not depression per se in a parent that is correlated with depression in a child. Rather, it is the impact that parental depression has on other, mediating variables. These include problem solving, affective involvement, and rates of criticism expressed that negatively affect an adolescent's well-being. These mediating variables are not specific to parental depression.
4. An underemphasized but notable finding is that depressed children or adults have an experience of their families that is at odds with that of other family members (Offer et al., 1982; Keitner et al., 1987). Although this may be a consequence of depressive thinking, the possibility exists that this dynamic contributes to depressive symptomatology.
5. The negative impact of disturbed family processes is reduced in the presence of a nonpathological parent (Valone et al., 1984; Hops et al., 1987; Jacobs et al., 1991). Having a supportive, attentive, low-EE, or nonrejecting parent represents a protective influence in the face of a chronically negative, unsupportive, or rejecting parent.
6. Causality cannot be easily determined. The most elaborate research designs suggest that interpersonal influence is bidirectional (Brunk and Henggeler, 1984; Tompson et al., 1990).

Most treatment models do include a role for the adolescent's other family members. Many clinicians see the family as crucial in helping adolescents recognize and alter their depressive cognitions, increase their pleasant activities, improve social skills, and increase self-control. Problematic interaction patters are also a focus for intervention. Clinicians and researchers have developed intervention programs that have been shown to be effective both alone and in conjunction with pharmacotherapy (Stark, 1990; Mufson et al., 1993). Future research on the families of depressed adolescents promises to better inform both intervention programs as well as therapy with these families.

REFERENCES

Alloy, L., Albright, J., Abramson, L. & Dykman, B. (1990), Depressive realism and nondepressive optimistic illusions: The role of the self. In: *Contemporary Psychological Approaches to Depression,* ed. R. Ingram. New York: Plenum Press, pp. 71–86.

American Psychiatric Association (1987), *Diagnostic and Statistical Manual of Mental Disorders*, 3rd ed., rev. Washington, DC: American Psychiatric Association.

Asarnow, J. R., Carlson, G. & Perdue, S. (1988), Childhood-onset depressive disorders: A follow-up study of rates of rehospitalization and out-of-home placement among child psychiatric inpatients. *J. Affective Disord.*, 15:245–253.

———— Goldstein, M. & Ben-Meir, S. (1988), Parental communication deviance in childhood onset schizophrenia spectrum and depressive disorders. *J. Child Psychol. Psychiat.*, 29:825–838.

Barnes, G. & Prosen, H. (1985), Parental death and depression. *J. Abnor. Psychol.*, 94:64–69.

Bifulco, A., Brown, G. & Harris, T. (1987), Childhood loss of a parent, lack of adequate parental care and adult depression: A replication. *J. Affect. Disord.*, 12:115–128.

Biglan, A., Hops, H. & Sherman, L. (1988), Coercive family processes and maternal depression. In: *Marriages and Families: Behavioral Treatments and Processes*, ed. R. McMahon & R. Peter. New York: Bruner/Mazel.

———— Friedman, L., Arthur, J. & Osteen, V. (1985), Problem-solving interactions of depressed women and their husbands. *Behav. Ther.*, 16:431–451.

Billings, A. & Moos, R. (1983), Comparison of children of depressed and nondepressed parents: A social environmental perspective. *J. Abnor. Child Psychol.*, 11:483–486.

Birtchnell, J. (1970), Early parent death and mental illness. *Brit. J. Psychiat.*, 116:281–288.

Breier, A., Kelsoe, J., Kirwin, P. & Beller, S. (1988), Early parental loss and development of adult psychopathology. *Arch. Gen. Psychiat.*, 45:987–993.

Breslau, N., Davis, G. & Prabucki, K. (1988), Depressed mothers as informants in family history research: Are they accurate? *Psychiat. Res.*, 24:345–359.

Brook, J., Brook, D., Whiteman, M. & Gordon, A. (1983), Depressive mood in male college students: Father–son interactional patterns. *Arch. Gen. Psychiat.*, 40:665–669.

Brunk, M. & Henggeler, S. (1984), Child influences upon adult controls: An experimental investigation. *Devel. Psychol.*, 20:1074–1081.

Bugental, D., Kaswan, J. & Love, L. (1970), Perception of contradictory meanings conveyed by verbal and nonverbal channels. *J. Pers. Soc. Psychol.*, 16:647–655.

——— & Love, L. (1971), Verbal–nonverbal conflict in parental messages to normal and disturbed children. *J. Abnor. Psychol.*, 77:6–10.

——— & ——— (1972), Videotaped family interaction: differences reflecting presence and type of child disturbance. *J. Abnor. Psychol.*, 79:285–290.

Burbach, D. & Borduin, C. (1986), Parent–child relations and the etiology of depression: A review of methods and findings. *Clin. Psychol. Rev.*, 6:133–153.

Cantwell, D. & Carlson, G. (1983), *Affective Disorders in Children and Adolescents*. New York: Spectrum Press.

Cohn, J., Matias, R., Tronick, E., Connell, D. & Lyons-Ruth, K. (1986), Face to face interactions of depressed mothers and their infants. In: *Maternal Depression and Infant Disturbance*, ed. E. Tronick & T. Field. San Francisco: Jossey-Bass, pp. 31–45.

Cole, D. & Rehm, L. (1986), Family interaction patterns and childhood depression. *J. Abnor. Child Psychol.*, 14:297–314.

Conrad, M. & Hammen, C. (1989), Role of maternal depression in perceptions of child maladjustment. *J. Consult. Clin. Psychol.*, 57:663–667.

Cook, W., Asarnow, J., Goldstein, M., Marshall, V. & Weber, E. (1990), Mother–child dynamics in early-onset depression and childhood schizophrenia spectrum disorders. *Develop. & Psychopath.*, 2:71–84.

——— Strachan, A., Goldstein, M. & Miklowitz, D. (1989), Expressed emotion and reciprocal affective relationships in families of disturbed adolescents. *Fam. Process*, 28:337–348.

Cytryn, E. & McKnew, D. (1980), Affective disorders in childhood. In: *Comprehensive Textbook of Psychiatry,* 3rd ed., ed. H. Kaplan, A. Friedman & R. Sadock. Baltimore, MD: Williams & Wilkins, pp. 2798–2809.

———— Bartko, J., Lamour, M. & Hamovit, J. (1982), Offspring of patients with affective disorders II. *J. Amer. Acad. Child Adol. Psychiat.,* 21:389–391.

Dadds, M., Sanders, M., Morrison, M. & Rebgetz, M. (1992), Childhood depression and conduct disorder: II. An analysis of family interaction patterns in the home. *J. Abnor. Psychol.,* 101:505–513.

Donenberg, G., Nelson, D. & Weisz, J. February, (1993), Poster presented at the meeting of Society for Research in Child and Adolescent Psychopathology, Santa Fe, NM.

Downey, G. & Coyne, J. (1990), Children of depressed parents: an integrative review. *Psychol. Bull.,* 108:50–76.

Dumas, J., Gibson, J. & Albin, J. (1989), Behavioral correlates of maternal depressive symptomatology in conduct-disorder children. *J. Consult. Clin. Psychol.,* 57:516–521.

Emery, R. (1982), Interparental conflict and the children of discord and divorce. *Psychol. Bull.,* 92:310–330.

Feldman, S., Rubenstein, J. & Rubin, C. (1988), Depressive affect and restraint in early adolescents: Relationships with family structure, family process, and friendship support. *J. Early Adol.,* 8:279–296.

Fendrich, M., Warner, V. & Weissman, M. (1990), Family risk factors, parental depression, and psychopathology in offspring. *Devel. Psychol.,* 26:40–50.

Field, T. (1984), Early interactions between infants and their postpartum depressed mothers. *Infant Behav. & Devel.,* 7:527–532.

———— Healy, B., Goldstein, S., Perry, S., Bendell, D., Schanberg, S., Zimmerman, E. & Kuhn, C. (1988), Infants of depressed mothers show "depressed" behavior even with nondepressed adults. *Child Devel.,* 59:1569–1579.

———— Sandberg, D., Garcia, R., Vega-Lahr, N., Goldstein, S. & Guy, L. (1985), Prenatal problems, postpartum depression and early mother-infant interactions. *Devel. Psychol.,* 12:1152–1156.

Forehand, R., Brody, G., Slotkin, J., Fauber, R., McCombs, A. & Long, N. (1988), Young adolescent and maternal depression: assessment, interrelations, and predictors. *J. Consult. Clin. Psychol.,* 56:422–426.

Friedman, L. (1984), *Family interaction among children of depressed mothers: A naturalistic observational study.* Unpublished doctoral dissertation. University of Oregon, Eugene.

Goodman, S. & Brumley, H. (1990), Schizophrenic and depressed mothers: relational deficits in parenting. *Devel. Psychol.*, 26:31–39.

Gotlib, I., Mount, J., Cordy, N. & Whiffen, V. (1988), Depressed mood and perceptions of early parenting: A longitudinal investigation. *Brit. J. Psychiat.*, 152:24–27.

Griest, D., Wells, K. & Forehand, R. (1979), An examination of predictors of maternal perceptions of maladjustment in clinic-referred children. *J. Abnor. Psychol.*, 88:277–281.

Hammen, C., Burge, D. & Adrian, C. (1991), Timing of mother and child depression in a longitudinal study of children at risk. *J. Consult. Clin. Psychol.*, 59:341–345.

Harris, I. & Howard, K. (1987), Correlates of depression and anger in adolescence. *J. Child. Adol. Psychother.*, 4:199–203.

Hass, G., Clarkin, J. & Glick, I. (1985), Marital and family treatment of depression. In: *Handbook of Depression*, ed. E. Beckham & W. Leber. Homewood, IL: Dorsey Press.

Hetherington, E. & Martin, B. (1986), Family interaction. In: *Psychopathological Disorders of Childhood*, 2nd ed., ed. H. Quay & J. Werry. New York: Wiley.

Hooley, J. (1990), Expressed emotion and depression. In: *Depression and Families*, ed. G. Keitner. Washington, DC: American Psychiatric Press, pp. 57–83.

——— Orley, J. & Teasdale, J. (1986), Levels of expressed emotion and relapse in depressed patients. *Brit. J. Psychiat.*, 148:642–647.

Hops, H., Biglan, A., Sherman, L., Arthur, J., Friedman, L. & Osteen, V. (1987), Home observations of family interactions of depressed women. *J. Consult. Clin. Psychol.*, 55:341–346.

Jacobs, T. (1975), Family interaction in disturbed and normal families: A methodological and substantive review. *Psychol. Bull.*, 82:33–65.

——— Krahn & Leonard (1991), Parent–child interactions in families with alcoholic fathers. *J. Consult. Clin. Psychol.*, 59:176–181.

Kashani, J., Carlson, G. & Beck, N. (1987), Depression, depressive symptoms, and depressed mood among a community sample of adolescents. *Amer. J. Psychiat.*, 144:931–934.

——— Orvaschel, H., Burk, J. & Reid, J. (1985), Informant variance: the issue of parent-child disagreement. *J. Amer. Acad. Child Psychiat.*, 24:437–441.

Keitner, G., Miller, I., Fruzzetti, A. & Epstein, N. (1987), Family functioning and suicidal behavior in psychiatric inpatients with major depression. *Psychiat.*, 50:242–255.

Klerman, G., Weissman, M., Rounsaville, B. & Chevron, E. (1984), *Interpersonal Psychotherapy of Depression.* New York: Basic Books.

Koestner, R., Zuroff, D. & Powers, T. (1991), Family origins of adolescent self-criticism and its continuity into adulthood. *J. Abnor. Psychol.*, 100:191–197.

Kovacs, M., Feinberg, T., Crouse, N., Paulauskas, S., Pollack, M. & Finkelstein, R. (1984a), Depressive disorders in childhood I: A longitudinal approach. *Arch. Gen. Psychiat.*, 41:229–237.

Kovacs, M., Feinberg, T., Crouse, N., Paulauskas, S., Pollack, M. & Finkelstein, R. (1984b), Depressive disorders in childhood II: A longitudinal study of the risk for subsequent major depression. *Arch. Gen. Psychiat.*, 41:643–649.

Lewinsohn, P. (1974), A behavioral approach to depression. In: *Depression*, ed. R. Friedman & M. Katz. New York: *Essential Papers on Depression*, ed. J. Coyne. New York: New York University Press, pp. 151–180, 1986.

———— & Rosenbaum, M. (1987), Recall of parental behavior by acute depressives, remitted depressives, and nondepressives. *J. Personal. & Soc. Psychol.*, 52:611–619.

Lopez, F., Campbell, V. & Watkins, C. (1989), Constructions of current family functioning among depressed and nondepressed college students. *J. Coll. Stud. Devel.*, 30:221–228.

Marriage, K., Fine, S., Moretti, M. & Haley, G. (1986), Relationship between depression and conduct disorder in children and adolescents. *J. Acad. Child Psychiat.*, 25:687–691.

Miller, S., Kabacoff, R., Keitner, G., Epstein, N. & Bishop, D. (1986), Family functioning in the families of psychiatric patients. *Comprehen. Psychiat.*, 27:302–312.

Mufson, L., Moreau, D., Weissman, M. & Klerman, G. (1993), *Interpersonal Psychotherapy for Depressed Adolescents.* New York: Guilford.

Offer, D., Ostrov, E. & Howard, K. (1982), Family perceptions of adolescent self-image. *J. Youth & Adol.*, 11:281–291.

Oliver, J., Handal, P., Finn, T. & Herdy, S. (1987), Depressed and nondepressed students and their siblings in frequent contact with their families: depression and perceptions of the family. *Cogn. Ther. & Res.*, 11:501–515.

Olson, D., Bell, R. & Portner, J. (1982), *Faces II.* St. Paul: University of Minnesota Press.

Orvaschel, H., Welsh-Allis, G. & Weijai, Y. (1988), Psychopathology in children of parents with recurrent depression. *J. Abnor. Child Psychol.*, 16:17–28.

Puig-Antich, J., Lukens, E., Davies, M., Goetz, D., Brennan-Quattrock, J. & Todak, G. (1985a), Psychosocial functioning in prepubertal major depressive disorders: I. Interpersonal relationships during the depressive episode. *Arch. Gen. Psychiat.*, 42:500–507.

———— (1985b), Psychosocial functioning in prepubertal major depressive disorders: II. interpersonal relationships after sustained recovery from affective episode. *Arch. Gen. Psychiat.*, 42:511–517.

Rie, H. (1966), Depression in childhood: a survey of some pertinent contributions. *J. Amer. Acad. Child Psychiat.*, 5:653–685.

Rogers, T. & Forehand, R. (1983), The role of parent depression in interactions between mothers and their clinic-referred children. *Cogn. Ther. & Res.*, 7:315–324.

Sanders, M., Dadds, M., Johnston, B. & Cash, R. (1992), Childhood depression and conduct disorder: I. behavioral, affective, and cognitive aspects of family problem-solving interactions. *J. Abnor. Psychol.*, 101:95–504.

Shaw, D. & Emery, R. (1987), Parental conflict and other correlates of the adjustment of school-age children whose parents have separated. *J. Abnor. Child Psychol.*, 15:269–281.

Stark, K. (1990), *Childhood Depression.* New York: Guilford.

———— Humphrey, L., Crook, K. & Lewis, K. (1990), Perceived family environments of depressed and anxious children: Child's and maternal figure's perspectives. *J. Abnor. Child Psychol.*, 18:527–547.

Susman, E., Trickett, P., Iannotti, R., Hollenbeck, B. & Zahn-Waxler, C. (1985), Child-rearing patterns in depressed, abusive, and normal mothers. *Amer. J. Orthopsychiat.*, 55:237–251.

Tesser, A., Forehand, R., Brody, G. & Long, N. (1989), Conflict: The role of calm and angry parent-child discussion in adolescent adjustment. *J. Soc. & Clin. Psychol.*, 8:317–330.

Tompson, M., Asarnow, J., Goldstein, M. & Miklowitz, D. (1990), Thought disorder and communication problems in children with schizophrenia spectrum and depressive disorders and their parents. *J. Clin. Child Psychol.*, 19:159–168.

Valone, K., Goldstein, M. & Norton, J. (1984), Parental expressed emotion and psychophysiological reactivity in an adolescent sample at risk for schizophrenia spectrum disorders. *J. Abnor. Psychol.*, 93:448–457.

Vaughn, C. & Leff, J. (1976), The influence of family and social factors on the course of psychiatric illness: a comparison of schizophrenic and depressed neurotic patients. *Brit. J. Psychiat.*, 129:125–137.

Weissman, M., Gammon, G., John, K., Merikangas, K., Warner, V., Prusoff, B. & Sholomskas, D. (1987), Children of depressed parents: increased psychopathology and early onset of major depression. *Arch. Gen. Psychiat.*, 44:847–853.

———— Leckman, J., Merikangas, K., Gammon, G. & Prusoff, B. (1984), Depression and anxiety disorders in parents and adolescents. *Arch. Gen. Psychiat.*, 41:845–852.

PART II

PSYCHOPATHOLOGICAL ISSUES IN ADOLESCENCE

Recent work continues to cast light on some of the characteristic psychopathologies of the adolescent period. Steven Jaffe updates the reader on issues in the assessment of substance use and abuse by teenagers, including some of the pitfalls into which the unwary clinician may fall. Further, he defines the necessary and appropriate treatment approaches to these difficult, if not intractable, problems. M. H. Schmidt and his colleagues report on a carefully designed and thoroughgoing prospective study of depressive and somatic symptoms in young German children followed into late adolescence. Schmidt et al. clearly demonstrate the predictive power of early frank depressive symptoms for later disturbance and, like Cantwell and others, find no support for the concept of "masked" depression.

4   ADOLESCENT SUBSTANCE ABUSE: ASSESSMENT AND TREATMENT

STEVEN L. JAFFE

Substance abuse is epidemic in our adolescent population and will be a contributing factor, if not the main problem, in 40% to 90% of teenagers seen by mental health professionals (Grunebaum et al., 1991; Jaffe, 1996b). This means that an understanding of what, when, and how teenagers use and abuse substances, as well as techniques for assessment and treatment, needs to be part of every clinician's training and knowledge. In this chapter, I briefly review some of the clinical aspects of assessment and then present a framework for relating specific treatment approaches to the level of substance abuse involvement.

Assessment

Alcohol continues to be the drug most abused by adolescents, with 35% of high school seniors having had a binge alcohol episode (five or more drinks on at least one occasion) in the past month. Marijuana comes next, with more than 21% of high school seniors having used marijuana in the past month during 1996 (Weinberg et al., 1998). If adolescents progress in their drug use, this sequence usually is from wine and beer to marijuana, to problem drinking, to LSD and pills (stimulants and depressants), to cocaine, and finally to heroin. One aspect of adolescent substance abuse, which is different from adult abuse, is that adolescents tend to abuse multiple substances. Thus, they continue to use those drugs that were used earlier in the sequence, although they do tend to have a drug of choice, the effects of which they value most highly. The incidence of drug abuse increases with age across the adolescent period for each drug in the sequence, except for inhalants, the use of which peaks in eighth graders (early adolescents). Marijuana addicts have described to me a drug use sequence that goes from cigarettes to a friend's or parent's joint, to beer and wine, to one's own joints, and finally to malt liquors and blunts (large marijuana cigars). Adolescents should be routinely asked about their use of alcohol and drugs. Evaluation will include exploring the amount, frequency, age of onset, types of agents used, and negative consequences. The times, places, peer use, mood, antecedents, consequences, and attempts and failures to control the alcohol and drug use need to be defined. Information from family, school, peers, and legal authorities is essential, as adolescents will tend to deny and minimize their use of substances and the ensuing negative consequences.

The clinician needs to understand the limitations of urine drug screens. A negative urine drug screen does not establish that the teenager does not abuse substances, although many parents would like to believe this. Most substances are removed from the body within 24 to 36 hours, except for marijuana (THC), which may be present in the urine up to 2 to 3 weeks, because of its fat solubility. Also, most teenagers know that significant hydration (drinking large amounts of water) will dilute their urine sufficiently to yield a negative urine drug screen. An adolescent who refuses a urine drug screen usually has something to hide. When an adolescent says, "Don't you trust me?" the clinician can respond by saying, "Show me" (Jaffe, 1996b).

Stage of Drug Use and Corresponding Treatment

As a result of the evaluation, the clinician should make a determination of the stage of substance abuse involvement. The following framework describes each stage and the possible corresponding treatment approaches (Jaffe, 1996b).

STAGE 1: EXPERIMENTAL, RECREATIONAL, OR SOCIAL USE

This is the beginning stage of use, with curiosity and doing what peers may be doing being the important factors. Teenagers often learn that drugs are fun and seek the thrill of doing something they are not supposed to be doing. They often find that use helps them gain acceptance by specific peers.

Stage		Treatment Strategies
Experimental use	$\rightarrow$	1. Education. 2. Counseling.

Treatment Strategies

For adolescents at Stage 1 (experimental, recreational, or social use), education and counseling are appropriate. Teenagers use drugs in direct proportion to availability and perceived safety. Learning about the realistic dangers of drugs and alcohol is helpful in these situations. For example, although adolescents tend to view marijuana as being a benign drug, the reality is that marijuana poses a serious threat to brain functioning, as it will decrease attention span, impair short-term memory functioning, and impair complex visuomotor behavior such as driving. Interestingly, impairment in complex visuomotor behavior is often not recognized by teenagers. Counseling is also needed for both teenagers and parents, as parents may need help in how to set appropriate limits with rewards and consequences.

STAGE 2: SUBSTANCE MISUSE

Here, teenagers are actively seeking the pleasurable experiences of using alcohol and drugs. Also, often they have learned that misuse helps them to escape from feelings of frustration, anger, depression, and inadequacy. At this stage, teenagers tend to use primarily on weekends, and there will be some deterioration in grades and conforming to rules.

Stage		Treatment Strategies
Substance misuse	$\rightarrow$	1. Education. 2. Counseling. 3. Individual and group therapy. 4. Family treatments. 5. Abstinence or "honest look" contract.

Treatment Strategies

At Stage 2 (misuse), in addition to education and counseling, individual and group therapies, family treatments, and an abstinence contract may be needed. At this stage, family therapies such as strategic, structural, systemic, and behavioral will be important interventions. Behavioral family therapy involves parent management training as well as contingency contracting. Here, specific, clear rules are established between parents and adolescents such that there are negative consequences to all drug or alcohol behavior or associated types of behavior and positive reinforcement of all activities not associated with drug use. Thus, positive reinforcement is given for going to school, doing homework, avoidance of using peers, and developing other recreational activities.

The abstinence or "honest look" contract is often very helpful. In this situation, teenagers express a willingness to stop using drugs and alcohol and to stop "druggie" types of behavior, and specific rewards and punishments related to this are established. Unannounced urine drug screens are also included in the contract. In this contract, teenagers express a willingness and a firm commitment to do without drugs and alcohol. Specific consequences if they are unable to abide by this abstinence contract or commitment are also specified, and these will include attending treatment at a more intense level of care.

STAGE 3: SUBSTANCE ABUSE DISORDER (STAGE OF HARMFUL INVOLVEMENT)

Here, teenagers are clearly harmfully involved and preoccupied with using alcohol and drugs. Drugs and alcohol are now being used during the week. The peer group is primarily a drug- and alcohol-using group. The adolescents know where and how to obtain alcohol and drugs and are increasingly involved in these activities. Alcohol and drugs are now significantly taking over their lives, and there are significant impairments in functioning at school and at home. These users have become very secretive, deceptive, and dishonest. *DSM IV–R* criteria of substance abuse will be met. These involve failure of major role obligations at work, school, or home because of substance use; recurrent use in physically hazardous situations; recurrent substance-related legal problems; or continued use despite recurrent social or interpersonal problems.

Stage		Treatment Strategies
Psychoactive substance abuse disorder	→	1. Education.
		2. Counseling.
		3. Individual and group therapy.
		4. Family treatments.
		5. Abstinence or "honest look" contract.
		6. Twelve-Step program—Alcoholics Anonymous (AA) or Narcotics Anonymous (NA)—self-help groups that "work the steps" and establish sponsorships.
		7. Cognitive-behavioral methods.
		8. Intensive outpatient, after-school, or partial-hospital programs.

Treatment Strategies

For teenagers at Stage 3 (psychoactive substance abuse disorder), a higher level of more intense treatment is required. Now, in addition to the education, counseling, individual and group therapies, family treatments, and an abstinence contract used in the earlier levels, specific treatment modalities and levels of care are needed. These will include beginning to work a Twelve-Step program, teaching of specific cognitive and behavioral methods, and attending a partial hospital or an intensive outpatient program. The partial hospital program may include a day program or daily after-school and evening programs or may involve an intensive outpatient program of intensive groups 4 hours every day.

Working a Twelve-Step program involves attending regular AA or NA meetings, establishing a sponsor relationship within that program, beginning to work the steps, and getting involved with a recovering peer group that is also attending meetings and working a Twelve-Step program.

It has been well recognized that adolescents, at this stage of psychoactive substance abuse disorder, will relapse, even if attempting to be abstinent, if they resume contact with their alcohol- and drug-using peers. Above all, attending AA and NA meetings and establishing social and recreational contact with other members who are working a good program are essential ingredients for adolescents to be able to stop using drugs and alcohol (Jaffe, 1992, 1996a, b).

Obtaining a sponsor involves the teenager's developing a Big Brother or Big Sister with an older member of AA or NA. The sponsor should be someone who has at least one year of good abstinent recovery and who wants to work with a teenager to help the teenager work the steps and deal with life in order to get off alcohol and drugs. Working of the steps is a core feature of Twelve-Step programs. Jaffe (1990) produced a workbook that is developmentally appropriate for teenagers to help them work their steps.

Step 1 is the most important, as it establishes the need to be off drugs and alcohol. The adolescents answer the questions in the workbook and then discuss these individually with a sponsor or a counselor. Then the answers are presented at a Step 1 therapy group.

The questions in the Step 1 involve detailed descriptions how the use of drugs and alcohol has put the lives of users at risk; has put the lives of others at risk; has affected family, school, and work relationships; and has affected self-esteem, mood, and plans for the future. Looking at the severe negative consequences of using drugs and alcohol helps teenagers to recognize that their lives are a mess on drugs and alcohol and that they need to be abstinent (clean and sober).

The workbook recognizes that teenagers like to use drugs but that they need to be clean and sober to have a future. The teenagers are helped to try to do what needs to be done to make their lives better and not what they want to do, which is to go out and use drugs and alcohol. Teenagers are also helped to recognize that they could not use drugs and alcohol in moderation and are reminded, again, of the need for abstinence. For teenagers, the emphasis is placed on becoming more powerful by stopping the use of drugs and alcohol and on the fact that this program enhances their power to have a life. Powerlessness occurs when they are using, and sobriety gives them power. The other concept used for teenagers is that, although it may be difficult for them to recognize addiction and dependency, they perhaps can view themselves at this stage of abuse as people who are on their way to being addicts.

Writing the answers to the Step 1 questions helps the adolescents to become more honest in acknowledging the extent of their use of drugs and alcohol and the effects on their lives. In addition to becoming more honest in how much they have used, the adolescents, in presenting the details of their answers in a group setting, often help themselves to become more honest with the emotional aspects of what had happened to their lives. In this situation, the defense mechanism of disavowal is undone, and teenagers emotionally recognize how bad their lives have become.

An example of this is the teenagers who casually and readily talk about how they had been on the street and raped when using drugs and alcohol. This episode seems of little consequence and affect, but, in verbally reviewing the details while clean and sober, individuals may begin to cry and realize how terrible their lives have become. Step 1 is so important because it is here that the motivation to be clean and sober is developed. Teenagers do not stop using drugs and alcohol unless they come to recognize cognitively and emotionally that their lives have become a mess and that change is needed.

Step 2 involves recognizing that they need to stop the insane ways they have been living, in which they have repeated self-destructive behavior over and over. The other part of Step 2 involves beginning to believe in a "Higher Power." This is a spiritual but not religious process in which the teenagers separate out what in their lives is under their control and what is not. They further learn that those aspects not under their control need to be turned over to a positive Higher Power. The workbook's approach is to first have the teenagers look at their childhood Higher Powers (i.e., the people who raised them) and to face the fact that these earlier Higher Powers often had neglected or abused them. Emotionally dealing with this grieving process then helps the teenagers to begin to look at something positive, greater than themselves, which can be the group, a positive force in the universe, nature, or love.

Step 3 involves making a commitment to work a program, and Step 4 involves taking a detailed moral self-inventory. Step 5 involves presenting the details of the moral inventory to a sponsor or therapist so it can be discussed and reviewed. Steps 1 to 3 achieve the adolescents' need and commitment to be abstinent and to work a program; Steps 4 and 5 help them begin to look at their whole lives and share this with another person who is in the program.

Important aspects of the Twelve-Step program include the facts that the meetings are free, that groups exist in every city in the United States and most foreign countries, and that these provide the teenagers with an abstinent, recovering peer group, which is essential for continued sobriety.

In addition to benefiting from Twelve-Step programs, teenagers at the substance abuse disorder stage are often helped by cognitive behavioral strategies that may be learned in individual or group sessions. These strategies involve learning specific techniques to deal with drugs and alcohol. Here, skills to refuse drugs, cope with urges, manage using thoughts, and handle emergencies and lapses are taught and practiced with role-playing exercises. Other communication skills, problem solving, anger and mood management, cognitive behavioral strategies, and relaxation training are important skills for these teenagers to learn. Cognitive behavioral skill training and beginning to work the steps in a Twelve-Step program are often part of intensive outpatient and partial-hospital and after-school programs.

STAGE 4: SUBSTANCE DEPENDENCY DISORDER (STAGE OF HARMFUL ADDICTION)

This is the stage of harmful dependency. *DSM–IV* criteria of substance dependency will be met. Usually, tolerance has developed. Withdrawal symptoms, which tend to be infrequent in the adolescent population, may be present. Attempts to control usage have been unsuccessful. Use of larger than intended amounts and failure of attempts to stop or reduce usage have occurred. Obtaining, using, and dealing with the consequences of alcohol and drugs have taken over most of the adolescents' lives, and they continue to use despite knowledge of the severe consequences. Addiction involves an inability to use alcohol and drugs in moderation. Adolescents at this stage of drug involvement might be able to have some periods of not using drugs at all, but, when or if they begin to use, the use rapidly goes out of control, with the return of severe negative consequences.

For teenagers at this fourth stage of involvement (i.e., chemical dependency) a hospital or residential program is often needed at the beginning of treatment. As they begin to make some progress in his hospital or residential program, consideration of a step down to partial-hospital and intensive outpatient programs can be made. In all intensive outpatient and partial-hospital programs, steps must be taken so the teenagers do not return to using peers, or else they will fail at that level of care. All of the previously described treatment strategies, especially the Twelve-Step program, are needed for treatment of substance-dependent adolescents. If a teenager fails at one level of care corresponding to a specific stage of drug involvement, this often indicates that a more advanced abuse or dependency stage was actually present and that the treatment modalities of this more advanced stage will be needed.

Stage	Treatment Strategies
Psychoactive substance dependency disorder →	1. Education.
	2. Counseling.
	3. Individual and group therapy.
	4. Family treatments.
	5. Abstinence or "honest look" contract.
	6. Twelve-step program—AA or NA—self-help groups that work the steps and establish sponsorships.
	7. Cognitive-behavioral methods.
	8. Intensive outpatient, after-school, or partial hospital programs.
	9. Hospital or residential programs.

Comorbidity and Pharmacological Treatment

Adolescents with substance abuse disorders have a high incidence (50% to 90%) of other psychiatric disorders, especially mood, behavior, and anxiety disorders (DeMilio, 1989; Bukstein, Glancy, and Kaminer, 1992). The specific treatment modalities described for the substance abuse stages are for the goal of abstinence from alcohol and drugs.

Parallel treatment of other coexisting psychiatric disorders is also needed. Successful treatment of the comorbid disorder is usually not possible if the adolescent continues to use and abuse substances. Treatment of the coexisting disorders is needed so that the adolescent does not relapse into using alcohol and drugs. Pharmacological treatments—especially mood stabilizers for aggression and bipolar disorder and antidepressants for depressive disorders—are often helpful. Of course, the adolescent's treatment compliance must be carefully monitored.

Conclusion

There is little research on specific treatment modalities with adolescent substance use disorders, and the efficacy of one treatment compared to another has not been demonstrated. Thus, a multimodal, multisystem approach that requires the highest level of the clinician's knowledge and skills is needed. Combinations of the treatment strategies described for substance abuse disorders are needed, as well as treatment of the coexisting psychiatric disorders. These need to be integrated into a multisystem approach in which problems in the family, school, peer group, and community are addressed. Although the pressures and challenges for the clinician working in this area are great, treatment success saves lives.

REFERENCES

Bukstein, O. G., Glancy, L. J. & Kaminer, Y. (1992), Patterns of affective comorbidity in a clinical population of dually diagnosed adolescent substance abusers. *J. Amer. Acad. Child & Adoles. Psychiat.*, 31:1041–1045.

DeMilio, L. (1989), Psychiatric syndromes in adolescent substance abusers. *Amer. J. Psychiat.*, 146:1212–1214.

Grunebaum, P. E., Prange, M. E., Friedman, R. M. & Silver, S. E. (1991), Substance abuse prevalence and comorbidity with other psychiatric disorders among adolescents with severe emotional disturbances. *J. Amer. Acad. Child & Adoles. Psychiat.*, 30:575–583.

Jaffe, S. L. (1990), *The Step Workbook for Adolescent Chemical Dependency Recovery—A Guide to the First Five Steps.* Washington, DC: American Psychiatric Press.

——— (1992), Pathways of relapse in adolescent chemical dependency recovery. *Adoles. Counselor*, 4(6):42–44.

——— (1996a), Preventing relapse: Guidelines for the psychiatrist. *Child & Adoles. Psychiat. Clin. North Amer.*, 5:213–220.

——— (1996b), The substance abusing youth. In: *Child and Adolescent Psychiatry*, ed. D. X. Parmelee. St. Louis, MO: Mosby, pp. 237–245.

Weinberg, N. Z., Rahdert, E., Colliver, J. D. & Glantz, M. D. (1998), Adolescent substance abuse: A review of the past 10 years. *J. Amer. Acad. Child & Adoles. Psychiat.*, 37:252–261.

5 PSYCHOSOMATIC AND DEPRESSIVE SYMPTOMS FROM AGE EIGHT TO AGE EIGHTEEN

M. H. SCHMIDT, B. LAY, G. ESSER, AND W. IHLE

Even today, when the psychoanalytic position that depression in childhood (i.e., before puberty) could hardly exist (e.g., Malmquist, 1971) has been given up, there are two approaches for defining depressive disorders during that age period: On the basis of an empirical study, Carlson and Cantwell (1980) criticized the concept of masked depression, which nevertheless has been held in serious textbooks (Graham, 1986). This concept proposed that classical depressive symptoms in children are masked by age-related behavior problems (e.g., hyperactivity, aggression and somatic complaints, phobias, underachievement, and delinquency). Ling, Oftedal, and Weinberg (1970) argued this position in dealing with the coincidence of headache and depression in children. It has never been clear how such masking symptoms could be differentiated from nonmasking disorders of the same kind in nondepressive children. Later, this position was dropped in favor of the idea of age-related "associated features" versus "essential symptoms" of childhood depression (Cantwell, 1983) under which somatic symptoms were subsumed as well.

More recent concepts have abandoned the idea of different symptoms in childhood and adult depression. But, in symptom lists like the *Diagnostic and Statistical Manual of Mental Disorders* (3rd ed., rev. [*DSM–III–R*]; American Psychiatric Association, 1987), somatic problems such as eating disorders, sleeping disorder, fatigue, and weight loss are included. The *Tenth Revision of the International Classification of Diseases* (*ICD–10*; World Health Organization, 1991) describes a special concomitant somatic syndrome. Because one of the best longitudinal studies dealing with depressive symptoms (Hoffmann, 1991) did not take somatic complaints into account, we followed this question using data from a German cohort study that independently checked somatic and depressive complaints at ages 8, 13, and 18. In this study, exploratory evaluation was done taking into consideration three possible relations: (a) there is no association between both kinds of symptoms at any age, (b) there is a continuous association between somatic and depressive symptoms, and (c) there are different associations at different age levels.

Subjects and Method

Out of a total population of 1,444 German 8-year-olds born between March and September 1970 and living in Mannheim on March 1, 1978, 361 (25%) were randomly drawn and asked to participate in the investigation. Out of these, 129 (36%) refused to take part in the study, and 16 were excluded due to low intelligence (IQ below 70), chronic diseases or severe handicaps, or because they had moved away from the area during the course of the study. The remaining 216 children formed the random sample.

Each of the 1,444 families of the initial population was asked to fill out a 40-item behavior questionnaire (an adapted version of the Conners scale) and to grant permission to their child's teacher to fill out the same screening instrument. After the random sample had been drawn and separated, screening data for 733 children were available. In order to increase the number of subjects with behavior problems, the most conspicuous 25% of the children with the highest scores in the teacher and parent questionnaire were selected. Together with the 216 subjects of the random sample, they formed the total field sample of 399 8-year-olds. Out of these, 356 (89%) could be reexamined at age 13, 340 (85%) also at age 18 (see Figure 1). Prevalence rates quoted in this chapter are related to subjects of the random sample. All other calculations were made on the basis of the total number of assessed children and adolescents.

Symptoms and child psychiatric disorders were determined by expert rating after a 2-hour parent interview. In the second and third stages of the study, case definition was further supplemented by an additional adolescent interview carried out with the 13- and 18-year-olds. All assessment decisions were made by child psychiatrists and experienced

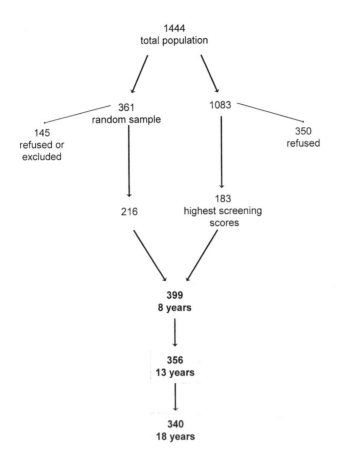

Figure 1 Sample.

clinical psychologists. Case definitions and diagnoses were based on the evaluation of 28 to 39 symptoms assessed as being *absent* (0), *moderate* (1), or *severe* (2), depending on the information provided by the respective interview items. More methodological details have been described elsewhere (Esser, Schmidt, and Woerner, 1990; Esser et al., 1992). Overall prevalence rates were estimated to be 16.2% at age 8, 17.8% at age 13, and 16.0% at age 18. In the original study (Esser et al., 1990; Esser et al., 1992), diagnoses were classified in four different categories following *ICD–9*: neurotic and emotional disorders (*ICD* 300 & 313), conduct disorders associated or not associated with emotional problems (*ICD* 312), hyperkinetic syndromes (*ICD* 314), and other specific symptoms and syndromes (*ICD* 307). In the present study, we summed up symptoms typical of these four diagnoses to sum scores.

Somatic complaints and psychosomatic symptoms were treated equally and thus were categorized in one group, but somatic complaints based on somatic disorder were excluded, of course. Due to the age-dependent developmental status, we checked for only 7 psychosomatic symptoms at age 8, 10 symptoms at age 13, and 11 symptoms at age 18 (see Table 1). The definitions of depressed mood and the various psychosomatic symptoms originate from the Mannheimer Elterninterview (Esser et al., 1989).

Results

PREVALENCE

The overall prevalence rates of psychosomatic symptoms and depressed mood are reported in Table 1. Figures represent severity levels

TABLE 1

PREVALENCE OF INDIVIDUAL SYMPTOMS

Symptom (Severity Levels 1 + 2)	Age (Years)		
	8[a]	13[b]	18[c]
Psychophysiologic headaches	22.7	49.2	43.6
Abdominal pain	27.8	30.5	14.9
Respiratory symptoms	2.8	7.3	3.9
Food refusal or extreme faddiness	14.4	24.9	12.7
Overeating	11.6	11.8	11.0
Anorectic behavior	—	.0	2.2
Initial insomnia	17.1	17.4	9.9
Intermittent insomnia	17.1	4.0	1.7
Hypochondriac worries	—	19.2	7.7
Abuse of pharmaceuticals	—	6.8	3.3
Somatization	—	—	5.0
Depressed mood	12.1	31.0	22.1

Note. Numbers are percentages.
[a]$n = 216$. [b]$n = 191$. [c]$n = 181$.

1 and 2. The two symptoms most frequently found were psychophysio-
logic headaches and abdominal pain. Depressed mood was reported at
each age level, with prevalence rates between 12.1% and 31.0%.

Table 2 informs about sex differences concerning prevalence rates.
Information is given separately for degrees 1 (*moderate*) and 2 (*severe*).
Most of the relevant sex differences were found in symptoms of moder-

TABLE 2

SEX-RELATED PREVALENCE OF INDIVIDUAL SYMPTOMS

Symptom	Severity Level	Age (Years)					
		8		13		18	
		Boys[a]	Girls[a]	Boys[b]	Girls[c]	Boys[d]	Girls[e]
Psychophysiologic head-	1	23	12	44	40	28	43
aches	2	6	5	9	6	5	11
Abdominal pain	1	22	23	24	35	11	9
	2	5	6	1	1	3	7
Respiratory symptoms	1	1	3	2	4	2	5
	2	1	1	5	4	1	1
Food refusal or extreme	1	8	9	20	27	8	13
faddiness	2	7	4	1	2	1	3
Overeating	1	11	12	5	7	3	5
	2	—	—	5	6	9	4
Anorectic behavior	1	—	—	0	0	0	4
	2	—	—	0	0	0	0
Initial insomnia	1	6	7	10	17	9	8
	2	11	11	4	2	1	2
Intermittent insomnia	1	6	7	2	6	0	1
	2	11	11	0	0	0	2
Hypochondriac worries	1	—	—	21	12	7	7
	2	—	—	1	5	0	2
Abuse of pharmaceuticals	1	—	—	5	4	2	2
	2	—	—	3	1	2	0
Somatization	1	—	—	—	—	3	7
	2	—	—	—	—	0	0
Depressed mood	1	12	11	25	35	13	24
	2	1	0	2	0	3	4

Note: Numbers are percentages.
[a]$n = 108$. [b]$n = 95$. [c]$n = 96$. [d]$n = 88$. [e]$n = 93$.

ate severity. The only relevant sex difference in symptoms rated *severe* (2) was found in "overeating," which was in favor of the girls. Overall, sex differences were more obvious in depressive than in psychosomatic symptoms.

INTERCORRELATION OF PSYCHOSOMATIC SYMPTOMS AND DEPRESSED MOOD

Table 3 and 4 show the intercorrelations of the psychosomatic symptoms assessed at ages 13 and 18 and the correlation of psychosomatic symptoms with depressed mood. As there was only one significant intercorrelation, figures of the 8-year-old sample are not demonstrated.

A comparison of Tables 3 and 4 shows that there is no special pattern of correlation between the psychosomatic symptoms, even if there are some more significant intercorrelations than expected at random. It seems important that the correlation coefficients with depression are at least at the same level as the intercorrelations. Furthermore, such

TABLE 3

PSYCHOSOMATIC SYMPTOMS OF 13-YEAR-OLDS:
INTERCORRELATIONS AND CORRELATION WITH DEPRESSED MOOD

					Intercorrelation						
	1	2	3	4	5	6	7	8	9	10	De-pressed Mood
1. Headaches	—	.29	−.04	.14	.15	−.02	.11	.14	.04	.17	.08
2. Abdominal pain		—	.02	.12	.12	.03	.08	−.02	−.03	.04	.10
3. Respiratory symptoms			—	.02	.08	.10	.06	−.01	−.01	.01	.09
4. Hypochondriac worries				—	.08	.09	.13	.02	.09	.18	.10
5. Initial insomnia					—	.27	.11	−.03	.19	.02	.28
6. Intermittent insomnia						—	.05	.07	.28	.08	.15
7. Food refusal or extreme faddiness							—	.35	.07	.15	.17
8. Overeating								—	−.02	.13	.04
9. Anorectic behavior									—	−.01	−.04
10. Abuse of pharmaceuticals										—	.01

Note. n = 356.

TABLE 4

PSYCHOSOMATIC SYMPTOMS OF 18-YEAR-OLDS:
INTERCORRELATIONS AND CORRELATION WITH DEPRESSED MOOD

	Intercorrelation										Depressed Mood
	2	3	4	5	6	7	8	9	10	11	
1. Headaches	.10	−.05	.24	.20	.10	.18	.16	.12	.02	.03	.11
2. Abdominal pain	—	.05	.12	.08	.04	−.05	.08	.03	−.13	.04	.10
3. Respiratory symptoms		—	.07	.05	−.02	−.03	.10	.14	−.07	.16	.01
4. Somatization			—	.30	.11	.05	.10	−.04	.07	.12	.29
5. Hypochondriac worries				—	.13	.07	.04	−.05	.00	.10	.15
6. Initial insomnia					—	.17	.05	−.01	−.06	−.03	.34
7. Intermittent insomnia						—	.10	.16	−.05	−.02	.17
8. Food refusal or extreme faddiness							—	.30	.02	.01	.24
9. Anorectic behavior								—	−.05	−.02	.15
10. Overeating									—	.06	−.06
11. Abuse of pharmaceuticals										—	−.03

Note. n = 335.

problems as falling asleep and food refusal are significantly correlated at both age levels with depressed mood.

SIGNIFICANCE OF DEPRESSIVE AND PSYCHOSOMATIC SYMPTOMS FOR PSYCHIATRIC DISORDER OCCURRING AT THE SAME TIME

Using odds-ratios, Table 5 demonstrates the age-specific role of symptoms for psychiatric disorder at respective age. A convergence toward the 18-year-olds can be stated that makes certain psychosomatic symptoms more meaningful. In contrast, even in 8-year-olds, depressed mood is of significance for psychiatric problems at that age.

By means of correlation analysis, we examined whether the sum of all psychosomatic symptoms is a more powerful indicator of psychiatric disorder than single symptoms at the same age. Table 6 shows that psychosomatic symptoms at age 8, even if more highly correlated with

TABLE 5

PSYCHOSOMATIC SYMPTOMS FROM AGE 8 TO AGE 18: AGE-SPECIFIC SIGNIFICANCE
OF SYMPTOMS FOR SIMULTANEOUS PSYCHIATRIC DISORDER (ODDS RATIOS)

	Age (Years)		
Symptom	8	13	18
Psychophysiologic headaches	2.4	1.9	2.3
Abdominal pain	2.0	2.2	1.8
Respiratory symptoms	1.2	3.0	2.9
Food refusal or extreme faddiness	2.3	2.0	2.2
Overeating	0.4	1.7	1.4
Anorectic behavior	—	3.5	5.1
Initial insomnia	1.4	3.7	3.7
Intermittent insomnia	—	7.4	9.7
Hypochondriac worries	—	1.9	5.5
Abuse of pharmaceuticals	—	2.4	2.2
Somatization	—	—	11.3
Depressed mood	6.0	3.9	5.4

TABLE 6

CORRELATION BETWEEN SUM OF PSYCHOSOMATIC SYMPTOMS, DEPRESSED MOOD,
AND OTHER PSYCHIATRIC DISORDERS (SYMPTOM SUM SCORES)

Age (Years)			Symptoms Of			
			Conduct Disorder	Hyper-kinetic Disorder	Emotional Disorder	Specific Syndromes
8	.15 {	Psychosomatic symptoms	.03	.12	.20	.06
		Depressed mood	.18	.19	.24	.20
13	.25 {	Psychosomatic symptoms	.25	.21	.43	.23
		Depressed mood	.11	.08	.39	.03
18	.33 {	Psychosomatic symptoms	.20	.32	.34	.17
		Depressed mood	.10	.12	.42	.01

Note. Correlation $\geq .17 : p < .001.$

internalizing symptoms, are fairly meaningless. Their value increases by ages 13 and 18—of course, mostly for internalizing symptoms. In contrast, the widespread significance of depression at age 8 concentrates on correlations with internalizing symptoms at ages 13 and 18.

STABILITY OF SYMPTOMS

Analyzing the longitudinal data, the specific issues to be investigated included the persistence of symptoms. Table 7 shows in what percentage certain symptoms occurring at a certain age could still be found at a later assessment. For example, in 73.3% of the 8-year-olds with headaches, headaches were still reported at age 13. Of course, the stability for the 10-year interval is lower than that for the 5-year interval. Keeping in mind the expected decrease, the symptoms of headache, overeating, and initial insomnias show remarkable stability. Further, the stability of these symptoms from age 8 to age 13 is similar to that from age 13 to age 18. Other rates show the decreasing importance of somatic symptoms from childhood to late adolescence. The high stability of depressed mood is noteworthy.

TABLE 7

STABILITY OF SYMPTOMS

Symptom	Assessment Ages (Years)		
	8 → 13	8 → 18	13 → 18
Psychophysiologic headaches	73.3	47.4	55.9
Abdominal pain	39.3	15.9	26.1
Respiratory symptoms	75.0	42.9	35.3
Food refusal or extreme faddiness	45.5	23.2	27.8
Overeating	54.5	54.1	63.2
Anorectic behavior	—	—	0.0
Initial insomnia	32.7	25.5	30.3
Intermittent insomnia	—	—	11.1
Hypochondriac worries	—	—	27.9
Abuse of pharmaceuticals	—	—	13.3
Depressed mood	45.8	33.3	44.8

Notes. Numbers are percentages. Dashes (—) = symptoms not reported in the same way.

TABLE 8

PREDICTIVE VALUE OF SYMPTOMS FOR PSYCHIATRIC DISORDER AT AGES 13 AND 18
OF CHILDREN UNDISTURBED AT AGES 8 AND 13

Symptom	Percentage of Undisturbed Children (Ages 8 and 13) Who Later (Ages 13 and 18) Developed Psychiatric Disorder		
	Ages 8 → 13	Ages 8 → 18	Ages 13 → 18
Psychophysiologic headaches	24*	19	16
Abdominal pain	12	23	9
Respiratory symptoms	33	40	10
Food refusal or extreme faddiness	14	18	17
Overeating	12	21	20
Sleep problems	16	24	13
Hypochondriac worries			15
Abuse of pharmaceuticals			44**
Depressed mood	28**	30*	19

Significance of χ^2: $^*p < .05$. $^{**}p < .01$. Comparison with children not displaying the respective symptom.

PREDICTIVE VALUE OF SYMPTOMS FOR LATER PSYCHIATRIC DISORDER

Table 8 deals with the predictive value of symptoms for later psychiatric disorder. Figures represent percentages of children and adolescents with psychosomatic symptom(s) and/or depressed mood but without a psychiatric diagnosis, who 5 or 10 years later are assessed as having a psychiatric disorder. For example, 24% of those with headaches at age 8 were diagnosed as psychiatrically disordered 5 years later. It is remarkable that only childhood headache and early adolescent abuse of prescribed pharmaceutics are of importance for later psychiatric disorder. Unexpectedly, childhood depression is highly predictive, whereas adolescent depression is not.

That this is not due to the insignificance of the single symptoms is evident when regarding the sum score of psychosomatic symptoms. This sum score of psychosomatic symptoms was compared with the symptom of depressed mood concerning the predictive value for later psychiatric disorder in undisturbed children (see Table 9). But, even the sum score is not a better predictor than depressed mood.

TABLE 9

Correlation Coefficients of Psychosomatic Symptoms (Sum Score) and Depressed Mood in Undisturbed 8- and 13-Year-Olds with Psychiatric Disorder at Ages 13 and 18

		Psychiatric Disorder At	
		Age 13	Age 18
Psychosomatic symptoms	age 8	.03	.07
Depressed mood	age 8	.12	.10
Psychosomatic symptoms	age 13		.06
Depressed mood	age 13		.10

CASE REPORT

The following case report demonstrates the development of early depressive symptoms from childhood until early adulthood and their impact on later psychiatric disorder. Anne (name fictitious) lived together with her two elder sisters and her parents in a small suburb of Mannheim. The psychosocial circumstances of the family were strained by chronic disease, unemployment, and, later, by the earning incapacity of Anne's father.

At age 8, Anne went to her third year of primary school. Her school performance was slightly below average; due to dyslexia, she received special tuition. In the lessons, she was very quiet. Her mother reported that Anne tended to hide herself away and to show depressive reactions (e.g., cry quickly) and that she often was teased by other children. Overall clinical judgment, however, did not result in psychiatric diagnosis (i.e., severity of problem behavior did not fulfill the diagnostic criteria of psychiatric disorder).

At age 13, the assessment revealed compulsive cleanliness, tidy-mindedness, and slight eating difficulties. As at the previous assessment depressed mood was also obvious. Due to overall clinical judgment, "suspectible psychiatric disorder" was diagnosed.

At age 18, Anne was still living with her parents. She had many friends and a permanent boyfriend whom she planned to marry soon. Her good secondary-school qualification enabled her to train as a decorator, which was her desired profession. After having changed employment, problems occurred, because Anne felt she was being harassed by her colleagues and superiors. She reacted with nightmares, psychosomatic complaints, weight loss (to 42 kg; height = 169 cm), and, again, depressed mood. Her fear of going to work became so strong that at last she quit the job. At assessment, she had started to work in the stocks department of a supermarket, so that she was employed below her educational level. At this age, she clearly fulfilled the criteria of psychiatric disorder: she was given the *ICD–10* diagnosis of adjustment disorder with mixed anxiety and depressive reaction (F43.22).

Anne's course of psychopathologic symptoms shows that depressed mood does not necessarily lead to a manifest disorder. Not until additional distress occurs do symptoms aggravate to psychiatric disorder. In the present case extreme fear of work and symptoms of depression and eating disorder were reactions to severe distress.

Discussion

One ought to expect that it is possible to estimate reliably the associations between somatic complaints and indicators of psychosomatic problems, which demonstrate more or less physical resonance to affective stress in our sample. As already stated by Esser et al. (1990) the influence of dropouts could mainly be controlled. A standardized assessment was used. Interrater reliabilities were found to be very high (Esser et al., 1990). The main problem of the present study might arise from analysis on the symptom level, not on the diagnosis level. A replication study on the basis of diagnoses has been started. Another source of error could be seen in the fact that the calculations were not carried out for boys and girls separately. Whether sex differences present themselves differently on the diagnosis level than on the symptom level is an issue for further research.

In order to determine the predictive value of certain symptoms, associations between somatic complaints and depressed mood were of special interest in our study. From the three possible models, that of associations changing with age had the highest probability according to our findings. This general result must be specified.

Until early school age, somatic complaints are seen as typical symptoms, but their relevance even increases in adolescence. Their association with depressed mood becomes stronger with age, whereas such an association cannot be seen in early school age. Nevertheless, single somatic symptoms show remarkable intercorrelations, but correlations with depressed mood are of at least the same significance. Associations are mainly found for somatic complaints of the "depression type" (i.e., eating problems, sleeping disorder).

Depression at age 8 proved to be a good indicator of psychiatric disorder at the same age, whereas only some of the somatic complaints—mainly of higher complexity (e.g., "somatization")—were indicative of psychiatric disorder. This was best validated for symptoms with longitudinal stability, such as headaches, eating and sleeping problems, and depressed mood.

The course of former psychiatrically healthy children and youngsters with certain single somatic and depressive symptoms developing psychiatric disorder at a later age demonstrates the long-term predictive value of those factors for later psychiatric disorder. Again, early depression with or without somatic symptoms was of higher predictive power than somatic symptoms.

It can be summarized that the typical coincidence of somatic symptoms (e.g., eating and sleeping disorders, psychiatric disorder) gains importance only with age, whereas depressed mood at age 8 already has a high predictive value. Therefore, our findings cannot support the hypothesis of childhood depression masked by somatic symptoms.

Summary

Out of a sample of 399 8-year-olds from a city of 300,000 inhabitants, 356 could be followed to age 13 and 340 to age 18. Half of the children derived from a representative sample, and the other half derived from a sample of problem children assessed by parents' and teachers' questionnaires. Rates of psychosomatic and depressive symptoms at ages 8, 13, and 18 were compared, correlations between both kinds of symptoms were calculated, and the stability of symptoms and their significance for present psychiatric morbidity and later psychiatric disorder were investigated. Changing associations were found between somatic complaints and depressed mood at different age levels, but our findings could not support the hypothesis of childhood depression masked by somatic symptoms.

REFERENCES

American Psychiatric Association (1987), *Diagnostic and Statistical Manual of Mental Disorders* (3rd ed., rev.). Washington, DC: APA.

Cantwell, D. P. (1983), Depression in childhood: Clinical picture and diagnostic criteria. In: *Affective Disorders in Childhood and Adolescence: An Update*, ed. D. P. Cantwell & G. A. Carlson. New York: Spectrum, pp. 3–18.

Carlson, G. A. & Cantwell, D. P. (1980), Unmasking masked depression in children and adolescents. *Amer. J. Psychiat.*, 137:445–449.

Esser, G., Blanz, B., Geisel, B. & Laucht, M. (1989), *Mannheimer Elterninterview (MEI)*. Weinheim, Germany: Beltz.

Esser, G., Schmidt, M. H. & Woerner, W. (1990), Epidemiology and course of psychiatric disorders in school-age children: Results of a longitudinal study. *J. Child Psychol. & Psychiat.*, 31:243–263.

Esser, G., Schmidt, M. H., Blanz, B., Fatkenheuer, B., Fritz, A., Koppe, T., Laucht, M., Rensch, B. & Rothenberger, W. (1992), Pravalenz und Verlauf psychischer Storungen im Kindes- und Jugendalter [Prevalence and course of psychiatric disorders in childhood and adolescence]. *Zeitschrift fur Kinder- und Jugendpsychiatrie*, 20:232–242.

Graham, P. (1986), *Child Psychiatry: A Developmental Approach*. Oxford, England: Oxford University Press.

Hoffmann, V. (1991), *Die Entwicklung depressiver Reaktionen in Kindheit und Jugend. Eine entwicklungspsychopathologische Langsschnittuntersuchung* [Depressive reactions in childhood and adolescents: A longitudinal study on developmental psychopathology] (Studien und Berichte 51). Berlin: Max-Planck-Institut fur Bildungsforschung.

Ling, W., Oftedal, G. & Weinberg, W. A. (1970), Depressive illness in children presenting a severe headache. *Amer. J. Disease Childhood*, 120:122–124.

Malmquist, C. (1971), Depressions in childhood and adolescence. *New England J. of Medicine,* 284:887–892; 955–961.

World Health Organization (1991), *Tenth Revision of the International Classification of Diseases (ICD–10). Clinical Descriptions and Diagnostic Guidelines*. Geneva, Switzerland: WHO.

PART III

PSYCHOTHERAPEUTIC ISSUES IN ADOLESCENCE

Despite the vicissitudes of the health care system, a major portion of most adolescent psychiatrists' working time remains devoted to providing psychotherapeutic help to troubled teenagers. The challenge of engaging, understanding, and communicating with our young patients continues to serve as a source of satisfaction, whatever the constraints under which, too often, we are obliged to operate. Philip Katz describes with great sensitivity the problems of establishing a working relationship with guarded, apprehensive adolescents—in particular, the need to protect their sense of autonomy in the early stages of the therapeutic process. E. James Anthony's account of the hospital treatment of a profoundly disturbed but extremely talented adolescent girl takes the reader back to a happier era when intensive long-term therapy for such children was readily available. Anthony's paper is of value, even now, as a demonstration of the skills of a remarkably gifted therapist and of the value of such experience as a laboratory for the systematic study of the pathogenesis and the intrapsychic and interpersonal dynamics of such cases. In the discussion that follows, Howard Lerner elaborates on some of the theoretical issues raised in Anthony's paper. Finally, Elizabeth Perl describes the dilemmas facing the therapist when confronted with a patient's self-destructive behavior and the need to recognize, even to respect, its various possible meanings.

6   ESTABLISHING THE
       THERAPEUTIC ALLIANCE

PHILIP KATZ

The establishment of the therapeutic alliance is one of the major tasks and one of the major challenges faced by adolescent psychiatrists. The therapeutic alliance creates the atmosphere in which patients can expand their capacities for insight and self-awareness, accept information and organization, and, through identification and/or transmuting internalizations, develop the structures necessary for coping with life's stresses and crises. The therapeutic alliance facilitates the exploration of the transferences and countertransferences that arise during the course of treatment, spurring the growth of the observant egos of both patient and therapist.

The establishment of the therapeutic alliance does not always start with the first encounter between patient and therapist. There is often a preset relationship that the patient has developed with a fantasied therapist. I would like to illustrate this point with three case examples.

Edwin decided that he needed psychotherapy early in his 16th year but waited until his 18th birthday to contact me about it, as he wanted to be sure that he could get the Canadian Medicare System to conceal its payments for therapy from his surgeon-father. During those 2 years, he had many imaginary discussions with me, whom he had heard of but never met.

Jack, 17, had tried for a year to figure out how to maneuver his father into ordering him into therapy. Although he felt he needed therapy, he knew that, if he suggested it to his domineering father, father would say no. He took advantage of a minor car accident to paint a picture of himself as a drug-abusing, depressed, somewhat suicidal adolescent. Father decided that Jack should go into treatment and called me about this "emergency," and I saw Jack soon afterward. I expected to find a hostile, angry adolescent. Instead, Jack arrived happy to be there, loaded with things to talk about, and, when we chanced to meet that evening in a restaurant, he introduced me to his friend as his psychiatrist.

Dale was a 16-year-old Aboriginal youngster who was described as being extremely violent and uncooperative. He had been charged with an assault, and the judge had requested a psychiatric assessment. I was asked if I would do the examination immediately and was told that it would take only a few minutes because he would not talk to me anyway. Fortunately, I booked the standard hour. Dale wheeled into the office, asked for a cup of coffee, and talked a blue streak for 90 min, during which time he gave me a mass of information about himself and contracted to come for psychotherapy. Months later, when we discussed what had lead to that unexpected first interview, he told me that, the night before he came to see me, he had decided that he was on the road to jail and that he did not want to follow that road to its end. He decided that he had to let somebody get to know him and help him with his problems and that he would take a chance on me in the interview the next day.

In working with difficult patients, it is helpful to remember that the patient who comes into a psychiatrist's office only occasionally resembles the description given by parents, referring doctors, social workers, and so forth. I had the experience of being on a Child Welfare Board of Review that assessed more than 400 adolescents, all of whom had been committed to a reform school. Almost invariably, it was our finding, on interviewing the adolescents, that they bore very little resemblance to the hardened, callous youngsters portrayed in the charts.

Hilda Bruch (1974) wrote:

Whatever he had heard about his patient-to-be, or read in the sometimes voluminous case history, when the first interview finally takes place [the psychiatrist] does well to remember that this is an occasion where two strangers meet, with both having to take the first tentative steps to learn to know one another. It is a time of mutual assessment. How the initial interview turns out depends not only on the patient and his problems, how he presents himself, how he perceives or misperceives the situation, but also on the therapist's openmindedness, his awareness of himself and his feelings and reactions, his confidence in what he is doing, and his sensitivity to the patient's need for help and understanding [pp. 2–3].

In the last few minutes before they meet in the first interview, both psychiatrists and their patients have fantasies about each other—fantasies that, depending on their knowledge of each other, generate emotions of varying degrees of intensity. These emotions are present in all therapists and all patients during those last few minutes before the interview and are remarkably similar. They each come with fear. The patient fears helplessness and loss of control over his personal destiny; the therapist fears helplessness and loss of control over the case. The patient fears a failure to get the help that is needed; the therapist fears failing to enlist the needed cooperation of the patient. The patient fears punishment for not fulfilling the requirements; the therapist fears legal difficulties for not fulfilling the requirements. They both fear the unknown. And, they each come with anger. The patient is angry at having to face the risk of humiliation in surrendering privacy; the therapist is angry at having to face the risk of humiliation should he or she fail to help the patient. Yet, in those first few minutes of the initial interview, despite fear and anger, the therapist must try to allay the patient's fear and anger.

Frieda Fromm-Reichmann (1950) wrote:

The psychiatrist should remember that intensive psychotherapy is a mutual enterprise, if not a mutual adventure, between two people who are strangers and who are likely to be as different from each other as are the average personalities in this culture. Yet, at the same time, there is much more likeness between themselves and their mental patients than some psychiatrists may wish to see. As Harry Stack Sullivan (1940) put it, "We are all much more simply human than otherwise" [p. 45].

It is essential that therapists be aware of their own fears—fears that they will be unsuccessful, that they will be embarrassed, that they will be challenged, that they will be frightened, and that these fears make them angry that they have to walk into that room and face the patient. Therapists must keep in mind that the patients are fearful that they will be humiliated and will not be helped and that the patients are angry that they must surrender their privacy and seek help from someone else, a stranger. Yet, therapist and patient, with all their anxieties, fears, and anger, come together because they both have the hope of getting satisfaction for their individual needs—the patient hopes for relief from his troubles, the therapist hopes for success and reward in his chosen profession. Establishment of a therapeutic alliance consolidates those hopes and thereby lessens the fear and anger.

I have emphasized therapists' preparing themselves before meeting their patients, because establishing a therapeutic alliance can often be derailed by a therapist's detachment, disinterest, insensitivity, or various other manifestations of underlying hostility or anxiety. Most adolescents who come to see a psychiatrist do so because they want help, and they are willing to overlook, at least initially, the therapist's clumsiness. But, in many years of supervision and consultation, I have seen several adolescents who needed psychotherapy and could have worked very well at it but were lost because of their therapist's malfunction.

I would like to illustrate this point with the story of my near-miss with Johnny, when I was a child fellow.

Johnny was 13 when we discussed the opening minute of our first contact, which had occurred when he was only 10. He had been described in the referral material as a precocious, bright youngster, severely neurotic, with high levels of anxiety and some depression. He was seated on a bench in the waiting room of the hospital's outpatient department. I walked up to him and addressed him in the way that I had been taught.

"Hi, Johnny. I'm Dr. Katz. I will be working with you. Would you like to come to my office with me?" Johnny stood up and took my hand, and we walked down the hospital corridor to my office.

About 3 years later, when we were terminating therapy and agreeing that things had gone very well between us, he commented that he never would have expected it after the opening greeting from me. I was surprised and asked what was wrong with the opening greeting. He asked if I remembered it. I said that I did remember it and repeated my introduction.

He said, "Yeah, and it took me six months to get over it!"

I was jarred because for 6 months he had done nothing in treatment despite major efforts on my part to get the relationship rolling. I asked, "What was so wrong with that introduction?"

"You were so damn patronizing! You put me in my place. You were the doctor, I was the patient."

Rather defensively, I said, "If it was so bad, how come you took my hand?"

"I was desperate, and I needed a friend."

I said to the now 13-year-old, "But the waiting room was absolutely no place to talk; it was crowded and noisy. What would you have liked me to have said?"

"Just that! Hi, Johnny, I am Dr. Katz. This is no place to talk. Would you like to come to my office with me?"

My fellow residents and I, in discussing this afterward, felt that Johnny was quite right, that the statement, "I am going to be working with you," did preempt the field and did imply that the power of decision was taken away from the youngster. For this sensitive boy, who had already been steamrollered by several events in his life, being presented with a fait accompli was not going to encourage his engagement in therapy. It took 6 months to convince him that we could work together.

Although the first few minutes of an interview are significant with all patients, they are particularly significant with adolescents, as many of them are struggling for independence, trying to establish an identity, and choosing their place in the world. They are particularly sensitive to any signals from the therapist that their powers of decision, their intelligence, and their perceptions will be ignored.

In general, however, the developmental processes of adolescence enhance the therapeutic relationship, boding well for the therapist's success. All adolescents, particularly difficult delinquent adolescents, are hungry for adult relationships—that is, for relationships with adults who are open and emotionally available, who are accepting and approving of them as human beings, and who will be nonjudgmental about what they have done. Our patients seek adults who, on looking at them, see not the "crazy" adolescents that their parents or parent figures see, the "disturbed" adolescents that the charts portray, or the "bad kids" labeled by society but rather their potential, what they can be in the future.

Also enhancing the potential of the therapeutic relationship is the adolescent's need of same-sex adults for identification (Meeks, 1990).

Given the opportunity for friendly, positive relationships, adolescents will to some degree idealize the therapists and identify with them. This potentiates the therapeutic power of the relationship and is particularly important in working with sociopathic adolescents, as it fills in the gaps in their superego.

In working with narcissistically disordered adolescents, one encounters a strong need for idealized parental figures who enable transmuting internalizations to occur (i.e., internalization of some aspects of the therapist selfobject). These internalizations then contribute to the structuralization of the self, resulting in increased abilities to cope with narcissistic blows, to tolerate stress, and to maintain functioning when they lose empathic selfobjects (e.g., the therapist).

During adolescence, one of the normative narcissistic developmental processes becomes much more important than it was in childhood. It is called the *alter-ego/twinship* line of development, and it is one in which the adolescent seeks in his feelings of alikeness, of sameness, of twinship with other members of the human race the security he needs for the furtherance of his development—thus the importance of the peer group to the adolescent. That process can also include a twinship with the therapist, and, from the security of that bond, the adolescent may gain the strength to let go of some of the narcissistic structures of his childhood and seek mature selfobjects rather than archaic selfobjects. For example, he may try to meet his needs for acceptance and approval by seeking in the world around him warm and empathic friends rather than trying to meet those needs by replicating his unapproving parents.

One other facet of adolescence should be mentioned. Adolescents find gratification in acquiring knowledge, especially about their own and others' psychodynamics. It gives them a sense of power, something they need when they are so disorganized by their own development and feel so weak. As being taught by adults is commonplace in their world, it is quite natural to the adolescents that therapists should teach them about their psyches, their psychodynamics, their psychopathology, and how to be their own psychotherapists. There isn't the subtle or not so subtle resistance that one finds in adult patients, who feel somewhat demeaned by having to learn about themselves from someone else. Notable exceptions to this acceptance of being taught are those narcissistic adolescents who still cling to their infantile grandiosity and experience any imparting of knowledge as an attack on their grandiose selves.

Thus, we see that adolescents need adult relationships for:

1. Acceptance and approval, which increase their self-esteem.
2. Help with developing their observing ego.
3. Models with whom they can identify.
4. Selfobjects who foster structuralization of the self.
5. An alter-ego/twinship relationship that enables narcissistic growth to proceed.
6. The setting in which they can acquire knowledge about themselves.

Another interesting aspect of our field of adolescent psychiatry is that we do not always know when we are having a first encounter with someone who may choose to work with us in psychotherapy. We may be doing some community service work, lecturing to a high school class, or just doing a consultation. An example of this is in the very interesting case of Tony.

Tony was 15 when I was asked to see him in consultation by the probation service. He had been in placement for a minor delinquency and was now requesting to go home. He was icy, cool, and reserved during the interview, but he made a good case for returning home, and I therefore recommended it.

I did not see Tony again until 6 months later, when I came back from a weekend holiday to find that, the day before, Tony had been admitted to hospital on a bad LSD trip as my private patient. His parents had said I was his psychiatrist. There was a police "hold" on the case. When I walked into Tony's room that morning, I found him lying on his bed in his underwear, refusing to wear hospital clothes, and seething with rage. He greeted me with, "When the fuck am I getting out of here?" I replied that I didn't know, that I would have to talk to the police, and that wouldn't be for a while, but I'd try to discharge him the next morning. The following conversation then occurred.

"Can I have my clothes?"

"If you get them, will you leave the hospital?"

"No."

"So, you can have your clothes."

"Can my friends visit?"

"If they bring you drugs, will you take them?"

"No."

"So, you can have your friends visit. I'll write the orders and see you tomorrow."

I left, enjoying Tony's open confusion about me.

Play is the language of the child, but adolescents also play out many of their experiences and conflicts. Tony and I had just played around with themes of authority, and the results appeared the next morning when Tony met me at the nursing station. He said, "I saw you walking up to the hospital." That was not the Tony I was expecting. I thought I was hearing a friendly overture and said, "Would you like to go for a cup of coffee?" He said that would be great, and we headed around the corner to the cafeteria, got coffee, and settled into an isolated table. As we were sitting down, Tony asked, "What do you think of acid?" I said I'd had several patients who had had good experiences with LSD, but many of them had also had very destructive bad trips, him included, so I thought, all in all, it was a pretty risky drug. He said flatly that it had saved his life. I said I'd like to hear about that.

He then told me that, when he was 13, he felt very uncomfortable at home, didn't belong, got into delinquencies, and wound up being placed with a priest who had several boys living with him. The priest was a terrific guy, and Tony was happy there at first, but then he began to get increasingly obsessed with the fear that the priest might want him homosexually and that he wouldn't be able to say no. He became afraid to go to the bathroom or shower lest the priest come after him. Yet, he knew that the priest had made no homosexual overtures to him or any of the other boys. The fear, of his inability to say no, finally drove him to decide to commit suicide. He was on his way to jump off a bridge when he ran into an old friend whom he told about his dilemma. The friend, who was an acidhead, told him acid would help him and gave Tony some, which he took. It was a nice experience, and Tony said, "Now that I was an acidhead, I knew I could say 'no.' " He didn't need to kill himself anymore.

I was now intrigued by this bright, sensitive boy and thought that therapy could be really helpful to him. I told him that, as a psychiatrist, I was in the role of an educated guesser—I liked to guess at why people did what they did—and I would like to guess at what happened to him. He said to go ahead. Using Erik Erikson's (1968) concepts of identity confusion, I said I thought he didn't know who he was, what he was, where he was going. Not knowing who or what he was, he felt that he couldn't decide anything and couldn't say yes or no. After he decided he was an acidhead, then he felt that he was somebody and had the right to say no. He was thoughtful for a moment, then said, "I wish I could have said that." It was a double-jump. He had not only looked at the content of the interpretation but at the process in which I had engaged. I came back with a response that implicitly acknowledged the quality of his response and that I hoped would lead him onward. I said, "Why aren't you on your way to becoming a psychiatrist, or a psychologist, or a social worker?" He said he wasn't impressed with the social workers and psychologists he had met, and he'd heard that psychiatrists screwed up their own kids. By the end of our coffee chat, he had decided to come for psychotherapy, which he did for several years, with very gratifying results.

Some points about this case:

1. I would guess that whatever occurred between Tony and me in the original consultation had some impact and led the parents to identify me as Tony's psychiatrist.

2. In his icy, reserved manner during the consultation, and then in his body language, behavior, and choice of greeting to me about when he was getting out, Tony had indicated that he did not want to discuss his personal affairs with me. At the time of the consultation and then in his hospital room, I accepted his position, and, in the play about authority, I indicated that I would not use my authority to lord it over him and that I was open to working things out with him. This had a significant impact on him and led to his reaching out to me the next morning.

3. Tony's overture—saying he had seen me walking up to the hospital—was not direct, but the decision to say that to me was a decision to reach out. On hospital wards, many requests for help come in that form. One has to be alert for them.

The cases of Tony, and of Johnny, the sensitive 10-year-old, illustrate the importance of the adolescent psychiatrist being tuned to issues of authority from the opening moment of the first interview. We are all aware of the adolescents' fear of being dominated by adults, of being helpless, and we know that it is their regressive wish to be taken care of that potentiates this fear of being dominated, for they vaguely feel that they must learn to take care of themselves, or else. They fear the guilt that comes when their pervasive sexuality invests relationships with adults, so they need to feel able to extricate themselves from those feared but desired relationships.

We must therefore indicate in the initial session that we will foster adolescents' independence by teaching them how to be their own therapists, thus enhancing their control over themselves and their lives. By teaching them about the world, we strengthen their powers in competitive and stressful situations, which is strongly appealing to them.

The therapeutic alliance is with the patient's observing ego, and the goal of teaching the patient to be his own therapist plays to the observing ego. Establishing the observing ego maintains the therapeutic alliance. In some cases, there is no observing ego to be found, and, in some cases, it comes and goes; the goal of the therapist must be to help bring the observing ego to life, to stabilize it, to work with it. Clarifying feelings, behavior, and experiences contributes to the growth of the observing ego.

The therapist needs to be alert to the adolescent patient's sensitivity to the therapist's grandiosity. If the therapist begins the first meeting with questions about problems, without taking the time to establish the patient's willingness to participate in the therapy, the message the patient receives is that the therapist thinks himself so wonderful that everyone will immediately want to work with him. If the therapist is annoyed because the patient will not answer some questions, the patient resents the therapist's feeling of being entitled to have what he wants. If the therapist takes the stand that he knows what something means—a dream, a fear, or a statement, the patient will resent the therapist's acting as if he knows everything. I like to use my role as an educated guesser—I know several reasons why something occurs, and I would like to see if any of them fit, or if the patient has a better suggestion. We work together.

Therapists should also be wary of being caught up by the patient's pathology and losing sight of the whole person. There needs to be some inquiry about the patient's pleasures, interests, and achievements so that the patient does not feel dehumanized.

Let us now turn to the establishment of a therapeutic alliance with an adolescent patient who has a narcissistic personality disorder—a group that is comprising a steadily increasing percentage of our disordered adolescents. They tend to be quite grandiose, and the essence of their treatment is for the therapist not to confront them by interpretation or action but to build a therapeutic environment, a holding environment—one that gives them a sense of acceptance and approval, thus enabling them to break free from their developmental arrest and progress in their narcissistic development. A controlling, authoritative interview is an attack on their grandiosity and imperils any future therapeutic relationship.

One builds a therapeutic relationship with a narcissistic patient primarily through the process of empathizing with them—that is, by verbalizing what we feel, sense, or infer to be their feelings. As they begin to feel that the therapist is one with them, sharing feelings and sensitivities, a therapeutic relationship can begin to develop. Drs. Gustavo Lage and Harvey Nathan (1991) wrote:

> In patients with neurotic or object-differentiated transferences, the therapist seeks to establish a therapeutic alliance with the patient. The therapist is a clearly differentiated object, and functions as a center of independent initiative. Where the patient has narcissistic or self-object pathology, the patient perceives the therapist to be functioning as part of a contextual unit. The therapist cannot be a center of independent initiative without destroying the perception of that contextual unit. This severely inhibits his activity as an interpreter, as a purveyor of ideas and perceptions. What is required is the creation of a therapeutic environment, a surround, in which the patient will grow and develop. A therapeutic relationship emerges in which the therapist will be perceived by the patient as being in three different roles: (1) that of an empathic, mirroring self-object so that the patient will grow and gain sufficient confidence to be able to depend on himself; (2) that of an idealized parent figure so that the patient will feel secure due to a merger with this calm, powerful figure; and (3) that of a twin so that the patient will feel that there is another one like him, which gives him a sense of completeness. As the patient progresses, and works through the self-object pathology, he will then become ready for the therapist to move from a rapport to an alliance. He will then allow the therapist to become an independent figure who can begin to work on the object-differentiated pathology [p. 60].

A narcissistic personality disorder is often not discernible at the initial visit. It may take some time before the symptoms emerge. Often, the first clue to its presence is in the nature of the developing transference, where the therapist senses that he is important to the patient, yet the patient does not treat him as if he were a real person with a life outside the therapy.

Given that (a) one can not always see evidence of a narcissistic personality disorder at the beginning of treatment, (b) narcissistic personality disorders constitute a significant portion of the adolescent psychiatric population, (c) interpretation and confrontation are contraindicated in the early stages of the treatment of narcissistic personality disorders, and (d) there are narcissistic elements in all patients, isn't it logical that we should use a gentle empathic approach at the beginning of treatment of all our patients? I have found this style of approach very helpful in engaging many difficult adolescents in therapy, whether they were narcissistic personality disorders or not.

I have mentioned that interpretation and confrontation are contraindicated early in the treatment of narcissistic personality disorders because they imply that there is something wrong with the patient. As these patients very frequently are quite grandiose, that implication is experienced as an attack on them, which is destructive to the therapeutic relationship. Tarachow (1963) pointed out that, even in neurotic patients, interpretations result in an object loss that, in order for the treatment to be successful, must be replaced with another object, the sympathetic therapist.

Throughout the literature, there are constant cautions against overuse and hasty use of interpretations, dating back to Sigmund Freud, whom Frieda Fromm-Reichmann (1950) quoted as saying, "The psychoanalyst's job is to help the patient, not to demonstrate how clever the doctor is" (p. 19).

Another of the areas in which there is a sharp differentiation in the early stages of treatment is the management of the idealization of the therapist. In the treatment of neurotic patients, one tends to reality-test their idealized image of the therapist; with narcissistic personality disorder patients, one accepts the idealization as something they need in order to feel secure enough to progress in their development. Dr. Lage likes to say that adolescent patients do not come to the therapist because the therapist is some ordinary guy with problems of his own; they come because the therapist is the Oracle of Delphi, which has all the answers, and they need the therapist to be the Oracle of Delphi—to which one of my young colleagues replied, "I don't mind when they want me to be the Oracle of Delphi. I have trouble when they want me to be the burning bush!"

From the beginning of treatment, there will be disruptions of the therapeutic alliance, and disruptions will continue to occur throughout the course of treatment. The therapist's alliance with the observing ego provides the means with which to overcome these disruptions—by enabling the therapist and the patient to cooperate in working out the cause of the disruption, turning something potentially harmful into something constructive.

There are many causes for the disruption of a treatment alliance. The therapist is bound to repeatedly frustrate the wishes of the patient—wishes that may be unrealistic or insatiable. The therapist may fail to empathize with the patient's feelings, missing the significance of various events. The realities of the therapist's own life, sickness, having to move appointments, family needs—all may lead to problems in the therapeutic alliance. These disruptions are not necessarily destructive—they may provide an opportunity for constructive work in therapy. As Michael Basch (1984) pointed out, the therapist can never be all that the patient wants him to be, and he therefore evokes the original traumatic condition. The failure of the therapist to be a libidinal object in transference neurosis, or to be a selfobject in the treatment of self-pathology, results in a disturbance of the treatment. It is the resolution, the working through, of these disturbances that is the curative aspect of treatment.

What about the adolescent who does not want any part of the therapist, let alone establish a therapeutic alliance?

Elsewhere (Katz, 1990), I have stated that there was a need for the therapist to have an armamentarium of strategies ready and available for instant use in the opening minutes of the first interview, and I suggested four such strategies for engaging the difficult adolescent:

1. Acknowledge your role as a stranger, saying that you do not expect the patient to trust you, he doesn't know you, you are a stranger. Invite the patient to try you out and see whether he or she would like to work with you. Verbalizing the thoughts that are already uppermost in the patient's mind shows the patient that the psychiatrist has possibilities for understanding him. The psychiatrist's acceptance that he has to prove himself to the patient protects the psychiatrist, a bit, from the powerful negative reactions that the patient has already built up against authority figures. It recognizes the patient's position of control. There is an implicit acceptance of the patient's intelligence and ability to

make good decisions. This is particularly helpful with difficult patients from a different ethnic background.

2. Seek opportunities to empathize, to show that you are trying to understand the patient's situation.

3. Analyze the situation to the patient and seek his or her assistance in working it out. I have a favorite example for demonstrating this technique.

Perry was a sixteen-year-old foster child who had recently become severely depressed. He had broken up with his girlfriend, was making a mess of his schooling, had become very difficult to live with in the foster home, and was engaging in some delinquent activities. The agency had been unable to work with him, and he was refusing to see any therapist. I suggested that they order him to see me once, telling him that he had to come one time but that they would not make him come more than that.

Perry slipped past the secretary and booted open the door to my agency office. He slammed into a chair and glared at me. I said, "You think you have it so bad! How would you like to be me, facing you? What would you do, Perry, if you were a psychiatrist and a social worker came to you saying that she had this very bright 16-year-old who is going to hell, who is screwing up his school, who is screwing up at the foster home, who has broken up with a real nice girlfriend, who is doing delinquent things, and is getting more and more depressed, but he is refusing to see a psychiatrist? You feel that you would like to try to help him, but you do not know how to get him to give you a try. He does not know you, and he does not know what you are like. If you were me, Perry, how would you get you to give me a try?"

He looked at me with a faint smile, was thoughtful for a few moments, and then said, "I don't know, but I'll give you a try."

In planning this approach, I had thought, from the description I had been given of the youngster as someone who was bright, thoughtful, and sensitive, that he would be intrigued by my approach. We went on from that beginning to a successful course of treatment.

4. Seek opportunities to offer help, to give concrete evidence of your interest in helping.

Remember that adolescents talk with their feet; whatever they may say, if they come to the sessions, there is some part of themselves, an observant ego, that is willing to try psychotherapy.

What about the goals of therapy? Galatzer-Levy (1991) wrote:

The central goal of adolescent psychotherapy is to renew the adolescent's capacity to grow and develop. Health is the ability to engage in further development, not a state from which symptoms are absent. When treatment goes well, however, youngsters take away even more than the resumption of development. They learn something of how to approach and rectify situations that cause them difficulty later on. This capacity may vary from the largely unconscious ability to rework fantasies and aspects of the personality to simply taking away "words of wisdom" from the therapist [p. 86].

In some cases, one of the therapist's goals may be to provide, to the patient, during the course of therapy, what has been called "a corrective emotional experience," or a "third-parent relationship" in which the patient learns that not all adults are harshly critical or coldly ungiving.

I would emphasize, however, that the goal of psychotherapy, in the majority of cases, is to teach the patient how to be his or her own therapist, so that the therapist becomes unnecessary. In treatment, our patients must learn how to make decisions that are in their own best long-term interests. We teach them how to weigh the pros and cons of a difficult situation, how to look at all sides of a question; we teach them to distinguish between thought and action; and we teach them psychodynamics, what makes them tick, and what makes their parents and everyone else tick.

An example of a patient becoming his own therapist is that of David, a 14-year-old, with major narcissistic problems who had been in therapy for a couple of years. He arrived for a session looking rather disorganized, talking in a rapid-fire way, with the verbal content jumping all over the place. He didn't make sense. I had never seen him this way before. I gently said to him that he was hopping around too much, that I couldn't make sense out of what he was saying. He replied that several of his classmates had said that to him today, and he could see that. I asked if he was that way last night, and he said no, and he was not that way when he woke up. We traced the time of change to just after his arrival at the private school he attended, when he went to see his favorite teacher, who had always treated him as someone special.

This time, however, the teacher was dealing with a crisis with another student and brushed off my patient. It was then that David fragmented. As we talked about his unconscious interpretation of the teacher's actions as rejection, he was able to reality test it, and he quickly settled down and began to function in his usual fashion. Over the next few years, on several occasions, he reported that he caught himself getting loose like that, and he successfully traced this back to the precipitating narcissistic blow, with good results.

Finally, the therapist must always be cognizant of the fact that psychotherapy is not done to a patient, it is done together with a patient.

As Bruch (1974) wrote, "The essential task [is] to listen with an honest and open mind, to convey to a patient that one is available for his journey of self-discovery but with the implication, from the very beginning, that this can be successful only when both take part in the work of this journey together" (p. 18).

In summary, the establishment of the therapeutic alliance has been overviewed from its beginnings in fantasies preceding the initial meeting, through the emotionally laden moments immediately before the first meeting, and into the first meeting. There has been an exploration of how some of the developmental processes of adolescence facilitate the development of the therapeutic relationship as well as a review of some of the possible troubles a therapist could get into. I have tried to build a case for an approach to all our adolescent patients as if they all were potential narcissistic personality disorders, and I have touched on some of the special techniques required for this group. I have suggested a framework for setting the goals of psychotherapy, emphasizing the teaching of the patient to be his or her own therapist, to facilitate the alliance with the observing ego.

I would like to end with a quotation that I read a long time ago. It is from Sid Caesar, an American comedian, writing about his own therapy. He said that, before he went into treatment, he was always walking into darkened rooms and barking his shins on the furniture. Now, he said, the furniture was still there, but the lights were on.

REFERENCES

Basch, M. (1984), Selfobjects and selfobject transference: Theoretical implications. In: *Kohut's Legacy*, ed. P. Stepansky & A. Goldberg. Hillsdale, NJ: The Analytic Press, 1992, pp. 3–17.

Bruch, H. (1974), *Learning Psychotherapy*. Cambridge, MA: Harvard University Press.

Erikson, E. (1968), *Identity: Youth and Crisis*. New York: Norton.

Fromm-Reichmann, F. (1950), *Principles of Intensive Psychotherapy*. Chicago: University of Chicago Press.

Galatzer-Levy, R. (1991), Considerations in the psychotherapy of adolescents. In: *Adolescent Psychotherapy*, ed. M. Slomowitz. Washington, DC: American Psychiatric Press, pp. 83–100.

Katz, P. (1990), The first few minutes: The engagement of the difficult adolescent. *Adolescent Psychiatry*, 17:69–81. Chicago: University of Chicago Press.

Lage, G. & Nathan, H. (1991), *Psychotherapy, Adolescents and Self Psychology*. Madison, CT: International Universities Press.

Meeks, J. (1990), *The Fragile Alliance*. Melbourne, FL: Krieger.

Sullivan, H. S. (1940), Conceptions of modern psychiatry. *Psychiat.*, 3:1–117.

Tarachow, S. (1963), *An Introduction to Psychotherapy*. New York: International Universities Press.

7 TREATMENT OF A NARCISSISTICALLY DISORDERED ADOLESCENT: SOME THEORETICAL AND THERAPEUTIC CONSIDERATIONS

E. JAMES ANTHONY

Narcissism is a borderline concept that should not be used as a key to everything [Freud, 1914, p. 85].

The disturbances to which a child's original narcissism is exposed, the reactions with which he seeks to protect himself from them and the paths into which he is forced in doing so—these are themes which I propose to leave on one side, as an important field which still awaits exploration [Freud, 1914, p. 92].

Greece is a land of rocky ways, stony hills, and rugged mountains, so that the exquisite bloom of wild flowers comes as a surprise. Among the most beautiful of these are the *narcissi* with their glowing purple and silver coloration, and the ancient storytellers chose them to elaborate a variety of legends, perhaps the most poignant of which being that of Narcissus, the handsome adolescent doomed to self-love by the gods for misusing the nymphs around him—and thereafter wandering the glade around him, enthralled by his own reflection in the pool. Despite his self-absorption, the loveliest of the nymphs, Echo, continued to haunt him, but, unfortunately, she too had punishment meted out by the gods, so that her conversation was limited to repeating the last words of the speaker, which may have given undue and possibly disturbing emphasis to what was said. Other variations of the legend focused on what transfixed Narcissus to the imagery in the pool: Was it himself, the mother, a water nymph who had abandoned him early in life, or was it the identical twin sister who had died mysteriously under circumstances that hinted at sibling incest. What held one's therapeutic attention was the setting—the reflecting pool in the solitary echoing glade, with its abundance of imagery and seemingly constructed for the treatment of a narcissistic disorder.

"Original Narcissism" and Its Exposure to Possible Developmental Hazards

Primary narcissism, speculatively, has been thought to have its beginnings in the mother–infant relationship within the womb or following birth and breast-feeding or its equivalent and gradually or rapidly diminished by the increasing impingements of reality and separation. When the maternal tie retains its intensity or is disrupted prematurely, this can result in a significant interference with the emergence of normally ranging ideals, a sense of true selfness, and the coming into being of a distorting condition that Green (1983) refers to as a "negative narcissism" and a "psychic void."

There appear to be exaggerations of normal self-regard that are taken for granted and accepted as being in the nature of things, and S. Freud (1914), oddly, enumerated these as children, cats (all kinds), outstanding comedians, and human females, "especially if they grow up with good looks" (p. 88), all of whom demonstrate some degree of self-contentment, inaccessibility, and a need for being loved—a blissful state of mind much to be envied. Following Freud, one can refer to Her Highness the Adolescent Princess(!) in many instances. Loving others in competition with oneself comes hard to such types, as therapists find out.

Another potent developmental hazard comes from narcissism of parents who pursue perfection in their offspring almost relentlessly, overlook her shortcomings, and aim at providing her with a carefree life that will be much better than they had themselves and that, at bottom, is nothing but their continued search for their own "lost narcissism of childhood" (S. Freud, 1914, p. 91). Children of such parents often feel that they are under scrutiny and criticism all their young lives and may come to distrust and hate these prime "stage managers" even to the point of paranoia. Such caretaking perfectionists can give rise to tragedies that have been referred to as "Nobel Prize syndromes," fraught with disillusionment and disappointment. The self-regulation of self-esteem is no longer in the hands of the child herself and is liable to undergo wild fluctuations in the omnipotence–impotence cycle.

> The regulation of self-esteem begins to show a phasic tendency for the first time during adolescence. Not only is there a new upsurge of narcissism but also a corresponding sensitivity to the loss or gain of narcissistic supplies. . . . This bipolarity is kept within normal limits by the principle of reality governing the environmental transactions [Anthony, 1973, p. 228].

With narcissistic parenting, the self-regulation gradually gives way to the caretaking regulations until the rhythms get totally out of hand and merge into a less reversible narcissistic disorder. Bipolar parents are especially prone to disturb and distort the regulatory developments. The child who becomes ill under such surveillance has often been assigned a special role in which she was loved only to the degree to which she was able to fulfill the family ideals and aspirations by means of her special abilities; should she fail, however, she is seen as bringing great shame to her people (Cohen et al., 1954).

Another situation occurs when the child does fall narcissistically ill and enters hospital treatment, usually after some self-destructive episode in her life. The therapist is confronted by a patient whose intense egotism had previously protected her from becoming disordered but whose inability to form loving attachments brought about an increasing vulnerability. She presents as an attractive and articulate young woman with an urge to a morbid creativity that often exercises a powerful hold on parents, teachers, and eventually therapists who might all conclude that they have a budding genius on their hands. The appealing narcissism of the patient inevitably interacts with the counternarcissism of the therapist and, undetected, may bring about a narcissism–counternarcissism complex with all the pitfalls of a transference–countertransference neurosis but adding the dangerousness of an infantile type of self-regard, a reliance on omnipotent thinking that eventually fails to support the psychic structure and leads to a despairing disillusionment with the therapeutic process. An ad hoc workgroup came together at Chestnut Lodge to deal with the difficulties presented by such narcissistic adolescent patients and to research the paths that the individual takes in reaching the breakdown stage and in recuperating from it. The workgroup was thus seen not only as a supervisory force lending its understanding to the more obscure narcissism–counternarcissism complexities. It also helped to elucidate the possible relation of the narcissistic psychopathology to the third great upsurge of egocentrism described by Inhelder and Piaget (1958), which they see as one of the most enduring features of adolescence until the process of "decentering" makes possible the true beginnings of adult work, allowing the patient to undertake a real job and not bask uselessly in messianic aspirations. One further goal that the research team set itself was the theoretical welding of the emotional and cognitive factors of egotism and egocentrism in the emergence of the well-coordinated and productive mind able to subjugate its fantasies to the analysis of facts. Piaget refers to this as the stage of the "decentered ego" (Inhelder and Piaget, 1958), which relinquishes, to some extent, its "omnipotentiality" (Pumpian-Mindlin, 1969).

The Adolescent as a Model for the Study of Narcissism

Our initial task was to look at the prototypes available in the then long-stay adolescent division of Chestnut Lodge in the light of S. Freud's (1914) "third libidinal type," attempting to appraise from the extensive and intensive investigative material available on each case the psychodynamic factors delineated by them, such as the lack of tension between ego and superego, the absence of preponderant erotic needs, the disinterest in all but themselves and their own immediate needs, the high degree of aggressiveness as evident in acting out, the evident wish to be loved rather than to love, and the striking personalities that innovatively and often destructively affected their environments. As a group, we wondered to what extent we would manage to relate the adolescent Narcissus to the adolescent Oedipus and whether we would conclude with Grunberger (1971) that the two were antagonistic and that a possible therapeutic outcome could be, "Where Narcissus was, there will Oedipus be." We felt on familiar grounds with the short-lived oedipal process (especially in the female adolescent) before the mechanism of "removal" (Katan, 1951) came into operation. It was not easy to bring preoedipal and oedipal elements together at this stage, and we were inclined to agree with Pulver (1971) that, although the concept of narcissism was one of the most important contributions that psychoanalysis had made, it was also one of the most confusing. As a workgroup, we could also sympathize with Freud's feelings of vexation and inadequacy after his monumental struggles with his 1914 paper. His haphazard use of the terms *ego* and *self* did not help us resolve our perplexity. The current culture or even cult of narcissism and the public preoccupation with self-esteem and shame have highlighted the adolescent struggle, intensified the associated self-consciousness, and led to inordinate degrees of embarrassment and exhibitionism. It is therefore not surprising that we empathized with the description of adolescence (even before the advent of drugs) as a "perpetual intoxication" and that a treatment encounter felt somewhat like running alongside an express train trying to keep up. Winnicott (1971) clearly loved the nature of adolescence—its wild playfulness, its creativities, its "precious" immaturity, its idealisms, its immaturities—all of which can and do antagonize other worthwhile therapists who have lost connection and remembrance of their teenage years. Anna Freud (1969), who also remained in touch with her own troubled adolescence, could, like Winnicott, appreciate adolescent narcissism in all its exaggerations. She could even express concern as to whether, in any individual case, there was enough narcissism (from both primary and secondary sources) to adequately cathect the self, the body, and the psychic apparatus so as to ensure sufficient self-regard, self-esteem, and sense of well-being without the associated dangers of pathological overestimation of the self, undue independence of the object world, and persistent and extreme object choices. With reference to treatment, she points out that the uncovering of the unconscious runs so counter to the thrust of adolescent narcissism that the patient may be driven to resist any exposure to narcissistic injury that could result from the therapeutic inquiry.

Potential Treatment Problems as Reviewed by the Workgroup

The workgroup devoted much time to the difficulties inherent in treating the narcissistic adolescent. It was assumed that the patient would strenuously resist the assumption of patienthood with its implication of imperfection and that the weak and erratic object cathexis would make for a weak and fragile working alliance. The second assumption was certainly true and left the therapist somewhat wounded by the easy disengagement that could occur from time to time and at any time, particularly when the therapist was led to feel that some degree of bonding had taken place. However, the patients would often take to the situation with narcissistic relish, especially if they were allowed to control the transaction without undue interruption by the therapist. The more primitive the disorder became in its choice of defenses, the more difficult it became to maintain even a benign contact with the emotional life of the patient, particularly when sessions were overwhelmed by explosive narcissistic rage and a degree of unreality invaded the treatment situation and led to severely irresponsible acting out both inside and outside the therapeutic frame. At such times, the workgroup would counsel a transient focus on everyday realities, especially on any lapses (latenesses, absences, inattentiveness, etc.) on the part of the therapist, allowing such failures to be microanalyzed by the patient. It was thought that this transient reversal of roles would gratify the narcissistic needs of the patient and restore the balance to the proceedings. Asking for frankness in this supervisory process, the therapist was invited to be as stringently self-revealing as possible without actually taking on a patient role himself, although the group insisted that his theoretical assumptions, his technical innovations under pressure, and his counterreactions to the patient might be hugely informative about both the positive and negative impact of the narcissistic understandings and misunderstandings of earnestly conducted therapeutic endeavors.

The most conspicuous counterreactions at the start of the treatment centered on the studied aloofness and coldness of the patients to the "winning ways" of the therapists in their efforts to establish a viable working alliance with opponents (so it seemed) who chose to disregard the overtures or greet these with contempt or even derision—styles of interchange that were clearly well practiced in home settings and that reportedly ended in parental frustration and rageful withdrawal. For the therapists, the weathering of this cycle of depreciation and belittlement (alternating with phony acclaim and eulogy) clearly called for a degree of emotional resilience coupled with an independent autonomous self-regarding capacity. With some practitioners, self-confidence could be so shaken that they came disconsolately to the workgroup bearing raw feelings of incompetence and narcissistic pain. As members of the workgroup became more familiar with the double role of supervisor and therapist, their empathic sensitivities underwent a noticeable increase. In one of the therapist's dreams brought to the group after he had endured a particularly grueling session replete with denigrations aimed at his ideas, his deplorable techniques, and his total lack of understanding, he had the patient walking to the office door, completely cured and wonderfully grateful to him. He laughed as he linked the dream to his wishfulfilment and therapeutic grandiosity until the group pointed out the hostility in getting rid of this obnoxious adolescent and the way in which he had been caught up in what Kohut (1971) described as a "narcissistic web." There were other therapist complaints that were progressively treated more sympathetically by the workgroup as their own individual corruptibilities were exposed—the prolonged periods of passive reflecting and echoing in an audience role, the oppressive "know-allness" that interrupted any insightful contribution, the yearning for the more give-and-take experience furnished by the usual run of patients, the offer to "let someone else have a go" with an impossibly recalcitrant type of case, and genuine bewilderment at the unresponsiveness to his own heroic (perhaps too heroic) efforts at contact.

There were other negative indicators of growing mismatching— evidence of some blunting of the therapist's habitual perceptiveness leading to a demoralizing succession of empathic failures; a strong preoccupation with theoretical issues with many quotations from the literature in therapies that terminated prematurely; and persistent failure to grasp the obvious actions, reactions, and interactions at certain critical periods and instead to deflect his therapeutic attention to apparent abstractions that were presumed to emanate from the less conscious strata of the patient's mind. Associated with this negative indicator was the therapist's boredom at the superficialities offered by the patient that were condemned as "long gleams into the obvious." All of the participants in the workgroup agreed that an inward sense of care, contact, and a flowing communicativeness were positive indicators of an ongoing, mutual process.

The workgroup members, in general, responded helpfully to the process notes brought to them, but the apple of discord lay in the multiple theories that currently beset the field and bombarded the consciousness of the therapist at periods of vacuity and distracted him from his basic attentiveness to the therapeutic process. He would voice agreements and disagreements concerning the "Big K's" (Kohut, 1971; Kernberg, 1975), Grunberger (1971), and Freud (1914); note how adolescents made up for the shortcomings of mothering during childhood by evolving grandiose and exhibitionistic self-images or constructing idealized parental images; concern himself with the cohesiveness of the adolescent self; and preoccupy himself technically with the mobilization of idealizing transferences, mirror transferences, and the very rigid defenses against oedipal wishes. For Kohut (1971), the therapist should deal with resistances by providing large doses of approval during the working-through process, should keep a wary mind on being suddenly idealized and suddenly demonized, and always watch his own intolerance to the release of narcissistic tensions. Treating the narcissistic patient under the aegis of self psychology can provide the therapist with much satisfaction as he watches the patient's "growing self-esteem and realistic enjoyment and the unfolding of moderate achievement, humor, empathy, wisdom and creativity" (p. 199). It was not at all surprising that the workgroup was totally seduced by this highly sustaining therapeutic promise and equally less surprising to its members that, for the Lodge-type adolescent patient, Kernberg was better for theory but Kohut was better for therapy. Trying to fit adolescent narcissism into a tripartite or even Mahlerian model (Mahler & McDevitt, 1982), however, proved too taxing for the workgroup, which often fell comfortably into the topographical schema with an added touch of object relations. In happier times at Chestnut Lodge, before managed care, the patient could be seen as "interminably" as needed in a setting that provided individual psychodynamic psychotherapy, group psychotherapy, family and couples therapy (when needed), pharmacotherapy, psychoeducational therapy, and milieu therapy in little, family-size cottages all organized around a dedicated and dynamic staff (Anthony, 1990).

Case Example: A Narcissistically Disordered Adolescent Girl with a Bipolar Family Background

The prototype to be presented here presented on admission as a physically attractive, highly articulate girl of 16 years, independently minded, self-confident, and seemingly self-sufficient, meeting most if not all of the *Diagnostic and Statistical Manual of Mental Disorders* (*DSM*) criteria for narcissistic personality disorder. In the psychological evaluation, she was described in summary as "an intensely self-absorbed young woman with a rich fantasy life that included grandiose ideas. Simple solutions to her problems were not available or acceptable to her. She was easily caught up in complicated scenarios that she spun out in her head. Her narcissism interfered with any true reciprocity in relationships. Hypomanic defenses were extensively used to maintain her self-esteem, but her identity confusion, her emptiness, and her depressive concerns were all too apparent."

From a psychotherapeutic point of view, she appeared unrewarding as a patient, but, in view of our commitment to a therapeutic research study, the therapist, the director of adolescent psychotherapy at the Lodge then, decided, somewhat reluctantly, to take her for a patient, not realizing at the time that he was doing himself a favor in terms of a rich learning experience. He later learned from her schoolteacher that she was gifted and creative, a talented poet, a photographer with an avid interest in the imagery of the natural world, "but horribly entitled and seductively persuasive." On meeting him for the most part indifferently, she immediately asked if he could arrange for her to have a special kind of typewriter, as she preferred to type her poetry and have it look perfect. He was later to realize how intensely she pursued perfection in all her activities. When he appeared doubtful about procuring this special kind of machine for her, she began to coax him alluringly, without as yet really knowing who he was. He found himself wanting to tell her that he was the director of psychotherapy and not in any way concerned with finding equipment for patients. This reminded the workgroup of Freud's (1914) comment that feminine narcissism was particularly attractive to men (no mention of age!).

At this point, however, he thought it best to tell her that he was to be her therapist, to which she shrugged her shoulders noncommittally. It seemed to him that he could just as well have said that he was the clinic handyman with as much effect. Clearly, counternarcissisms had begun to operate very early in the treatment. Next he asked why she had refused to take her lithium medication, and she responded quite calmly that she would sooner die than put horrible chemicals into her body and that she preferred to live her life as naturally as possible. He said nothing to persuade her but instead inquired how she liked the Lodge and the room to which she had been assigned. What she chose to tell him was more surprising:

I look a lot at myself and photograph myself in the mirror; it's made me into a good looker, I mean good at looking. I am extremely perceptive of anything and everyone. As I was sitting in my room, a boy appeared at the window. I looked at his eyes, his mouth, the way he was holding his hands, his foolish smile and I said to myself: "I know he's been masturbating." I learnt later that this was true, and I was overjoyed at my perceptiveness.

This little vignette provided a good introduction of this prototypical case to the workgroup, and she was accepted into the therapeutic research. They summed her up as being grandiose, entitled, unempathic, exploitative, self-absorbed, attention seeking, prone to infatuations, and hypersensitive to criticism—which was the checklist taken from the *DSM*. Quite accidentally, she saw her diagnostic sheet and laughed mockingly at these "silly" assessments by "inferior, conventional people."

The patient was brought up in a manic–depressive environment in which almost every member of the father's family had manifested some evidence of the illness, including suicidality and alcoholism. At the same time, this was coupled with intense aspirations and drives to success. The paternal great-grandmother had hung herself, the paternal uncle had shot himself to death, and several close members had been hospitalized for affective disorders. The mother's family was equally given to extreme depressions and alcoholism, bringing together two strains of bipolar illness (Anthony, 1975). Both parents were highly intelligent and cultivated, with father achieving a prominent position in the media and mother claiming to be descended from Goethe, writing unpublished poetry at home.

So wild and weird were the childhood circumstances of these two people that they waited seven years after their marriage before deciding to have children, even considering adoption because of the strong genetic background. When eventually and unexpectedly mother became pregnant, they jointly and solemnly decided that they would give the child-to-be a growing-up experience that was quite the opposite to what they themselves had lived through. Mother later wrote about her infant daughter:

We knew from the start that we had a wonderful gifted child who had unique ways of looking at the world and would follow her own drummer towards her creative goals. We were prepared to give her all the latitude she needed in order to achieve these, and the best home and learning environment possible. *Our* goal was to see her go out into life with her spirit and talents intact.

116

It was a brave Rousseau-like attempt to create a utopian universe for their offspring, free from the usual and expectable frustrations of everyday life, in which a "child of nature" as they thought of her could very naturally evolve into an artist, poet, or writer but most of all into a "free spirit" unbound in any way by convention.

These best laid child-rearing plans of the well-intentioned parents gradually began to go sadly awry as their own disturbed and disturbing psychological histories began to catch up with them and impinge destructively on their creatively conceived lives. Elements of manic–depression entered the picture. The father suffered increasingly from psychosomatic complaints, becoming irritable, isolated, and often confined to his bed, narcissistically hypochondriacal and unpredictable in his behavior. The mother for her part reacted resentfully and depressively to her husband's unreasonable conduct, and, to make a dreadful situation even worse, the household was further disorganized by the presence of a volatile, explosive maternal grandmother who added her quota of unreasonableness to daily living.

The Rousseau-like child very soon began to show some worrisome behavior. As a toddler, she was fearless, a risk taker, as if the idea of danger was not yet a part of her thinking, and she would disappear from time to time roaming the neighborhood on her own and manifesting no apparent separation anxiety. Preschool highlighted her extraordinary autonomy. She constructed and spoke her own private language, even manufacturing her own little dictionary; she made up games that she played by herself and according to her own rules; and she would not adapt to any situation that required her to acquiesce to its norms. When she spoke in company, she insisted on not being interrupted. If anyone so much as touched her, she would state imperiously, "Take your hands off me; don't touch me; I am a princess and you may kiss my hand." She seemed to be living in an egocentric world controlled by an intense egotism. She did not reach out affectionately to anyone, although her parents were permitted, under her conditions, to cuddle or kiss her.

When the girl was four years old, a sister was born, and she underwent marked changes in her attitudes and behavior, becoming more unconforming and at times disorganized. She wandered off on her own, took people's possessions without concern for ownership, ignored her sister as if she did not exist, and worked by herself constructing objects that seemed to have meaning only for herself. She never explained anything. When she started elementary school, she was essentially a loner. Her peers avoided her, although she may also have avoided them. But, her teachers lauded her high intelligence, her creativity, and her unusual focus on her surroundings. They even smiled tolerantly at her unconventional conduct, as when she took off her dress in the classroom so that everyone could see her pretty underwear. Her parents still referred to her as their "creative butterfly," and it was true that she made an entrancing picture as she flitted from one interesting preoccupation to another.

By the time she entered middle school, she appeared to become increasingly isolated from the other children, often lost in thought and very much preoccupied with the film star, Marilyn Monroe—a sad and lonely narcissist if ever there was one, whose own beginnings were equally chaotic. She seemed profoundly identified with the star and would gather information about her and collect her pictures. She would frequently be observed sitting alone with a faraway look on her face, clearly wrapped in thought. Toward the end of middle school, she was no longer a creative butterfly but rather someone living in her own world and in her own way. However, she began making certain concessions to reality, and, although impulsive and ruthlessly unconcerned with others, she could become temporarily infatuated with someone—some girl, as she was at an all-girls private school—whom she perceived as being "sympatico," (i.e., just like herself).

It was in high school that her behavior reached degrees of outrageousness that made even her very tolerant school wonder if it could keep her. However, she made one or two contacts with "outsiders" like herself, and, at one point, because she felt deserted by her one and only friend, she cut her hand and smeared the blood all over it, causing a frightening scene. Things escalated after this, and, during a prom, she slipped away from the gathering, still wearing only a flimsy dress, and hitched a ride in the dead of night, in midwinter, from a trucker who was going to New York. Her intention was finally to reach northern New England and "live with nature." She had no money at all but carried her camera. (Photography was another solitary hobby of hers, relating her lonesomely to the outside world and its wonderful glut of images.) The kindly truck driver dropped her off at Central Park and gave her $5 to call her parents, which she did after staying overnight with a woman who found her on a park bench and took pity on her. She was returned to her home and brought hurriedly to Chestnut Lodge.

On her journey north, she had left behind in her room at home a few explanatory notes and several poems in the making. The first note said, "This is not my world and I didn't choose to live in it. I want to return to nature and live with the animals because they are the only ones I trust." A second note said, "I love all people and I will love anyone who will open their hearts to me. I always love people more than they love me. I don't expect to change and I can't change. The solution: I can only be happy because I love myself as much as I love me." This could have been the cry of Narcissus as he gazed hopelessly into the reflecting pool. There were two poems, also left behind in her Rousseau-like flight to nature, clearly written at the depth and height of her bipolar swings:

I can't escape from the silent
scream of my heart.
Why can't I turn it off?
I try to mute its painful cry
but it won't stop
my head roars as waves of pain
pound and crash
against my lonely shores.

Happiness consumes my brain
Tingling my cerebrum
Am I insane?
I'm in love with everything
Even the smallest clod
Of dirt in the road brings
Me to my feet to my feet
To applaud.

PHASE 1 OF TREATMENT: EVOLUTION
OF THE REFLECTING POOL AND ECHOING GLADE

As was predicted, the treatment began with intense resistances that seemed almost implacable. The patient could hardly bear to remain in the sessions and tried to find ways to occupy her time (e.g., connecting chains out of paper clips) but not without much sighing. When the therapist pointed out that she was not making full therapeutic use of the hour, she exploded with rage: "Don't you see I need to be free to roam wherever I want to go. You're tying me to the floor. I'm losing the golden minutes of my life doing nothing." She constantly reiterated that she was not a patient and needed no treatment or therapist. She was furious that he analyzed everything she said as if he knew exactly everything that was going on in her mind. She would never tell him anything personal such as her dreams, her daydreams, or her poetry. This is what the other kids had told her—"that you therapists try to squeeze things out of people." Nor would she ever show him her photographs, because he would not understand what they meant. The therapist responded mildly that all this was a big pity because he enjoyed looking at pictures, going to movies, reading poetry, remembering things from long ago, and daydreaming when there was nothing else to do. He liked all the images that walked around in his head. But, he had one big fault—he liked to make them all perfect. There was a long silence after this, during which she just stared at him without resorting to any distraction. And then she left as the session ended, seemingly somewhat reluctantly.

At the next session (to which she was early), she addressed him immediately, saying that she was very interested in what he had spoken of the previous day. As far as she knew, there was only one thing wrong with her—she was perfectionistic. "Being a perfectionist can itself be an imperfection. Try and work that one out. My photos have to be perfect, and my poetry has to be perfect, and I waste a lot of time making everything perfect. I also spend a lot of time looking at the mirror in the bathroom to see if there are any blemishes. I hate things not being perfect." (The cottage staff had reported that they suspected her of masturbating because of the long time she spent in the bathroom.) The therapist remarked somewhat tentatively that they appeared to be somewhat alike in this—that they both strove for perfection but often had trouble finding it. He continued, a little teasingly, that they might be able to help each other about this, and she smiled—her first engaging smile. This rapidly gave place to a frown. She abhorred the fact that therapists obtained information from school and cottage staff. "You must work only with what I bring to you, and, if I choose to bring nothing, that's just too bad for you." The therapist nodded his agreement and stated that he would try and keep his ears shut to outside rumor, especially because he liked the thought that this was to be just something between her and him "in our little neck of the woods," where they could just share their way of seeing and understanding things. She looked at him suspiciously and said that she could not recall their agreeing to anything. "I simply don't want people getting into my personal business." A rumor did come up from the cottage that her peers were becoming exasperated with her "playing the therapist" with them while resolutely denying she had any problems of her own. They also objected to her "queenly" insistence that "everything should go her way."

THE WAY IN: SHARING IMAGERY AND POSSIBLY IDEAS

The technical question arising in the "therapeutic glade" was how to become a mirroring therapist who could allow himself to be cathected narcissistically, permit himself to be made use of as any disposable object, increasingly sensitize himself empathically to the self-feelings emanating from the patient, and attempt to meet the narcissistic patient's implicit belief that the therapist should obey her as did her right arm (Kohut, 1971). At times, it could feel like being in a cage with a lioness who was also a lion tamer, with himself as audience trying hard to recreate the reflecting pool and echoing glade where strong feline aggressiveness would seem to be out of place. And yet, the patient's aggressiveness was becoming more blatantly manifested as the treatment progressed.

The therapist had the uneasy feeling that the situation was building up into some sort of challenge. The patient asked him one day to watch a video movie, *A Clockwork Orange*, giving three reasons. First, the video was one of her most precious possessions, and she watched it whenever she could, but the authorities would not permit her to show it in the cottage. Second, her father, "that dull, dreary, depressed man," had adamantly refused to watch it with her because, he said, its egotism, its sadism, its teenage violence, and its gross sexuality disgusted him (which were also all the reasons that delighted her). Third, if the therapist really and truly wished to learn about her, he might be able to do so by sharing the experience with her. The invitation sounded challenging, seductive, and transferential. The therapist felt that he was being put to the test but was not quite sure what he was being tested about or how the test information would be used for or against the therapy. However, the fact that it was his idea of experiencing imagery mutually led to his agreeing to "try the experiment." She took up a position behind him in the darkened room looking at the screen and, after the showing was over, said, somewhat factually, "I know which parts you found ugly because you shifted around in your chair," suggesting that her observing ego was honing itself on his psyche.

From images in movies, we turned to imagery in literature and read parts to each other of the Chestnut Lodge book, *I Never Promised You a Rose Garden* (her choice). She wondered whether that was what psychotherapy really was about. "It must be wonderful to have someone *really* understand you like that!" Perhaps being a man, and being old, and being a foreigner would make it quite impossible in this situation. The therapist pointed out that Dr. Frieda Fromm-Reichman in the book was old and a foreigner but understood her patient very well. The patient wondered if the therapist would write a book about her or she about him, and he said that, in either case, it would be about two people and how they worked with each other, not about one person. She began to consider the pseudonym that would be used for her in the therapist's book. Her own preference would be for "Pandora Peterkin," which would conceal the name of her favorite literary character, Peter Pan, the boy who did not want to grow up. She thought she was at her best when she was young and something of a genius, but she felt less of a genius now. Continuing with her therapeutic analysis, she wanted the therapist to know that *Peterkin* meant "little penis," which was how she thought of boys who were too chicken to engage in deep conversations with her; all they could think about was sex, which she thought was "so limited." She hoped that, in the therapist's book, he would emphasize her uniqueness, that he had never met anyone quite like her, and that, when she walked through any group of people, she would get stares and glares because of her outlandish clothes, her black boots, and her black nail polish, all personifying evil, although she was in fact nothing of the kind.

As she spoke, the therapist became aware how very young, naive, and innocent she was, although, in the hospital milieu, she was a perpetual source of disorder and disturbance, running away periodically, getting drunk in public places, shoplifting (because she believed in communal possessions—that everything belonged to everyone), using drugs, and playing Russian roulette with quite dangerous stakes. The authorities labeled her an attention seeker and a trouble maker. "I climb as high as I can, and I call out as loudly as I can, but no one in the world seems to hear me." The sense of aloneness was overpowering, and her desperate search for mirrored and magical love only brought her face to face with her own unlovableness. Pursuing images in her quest for absolute self-fulfillment only accentuated her feelings of total abandonment. She began to wonder whether her next step downward would be to a state hospital. "Would you miss me?" she asked the therapist bleakly but stopped him from answering.

MUTUAL IMAGERY BEGINS TO AFFECT
THE TRANSFERENCE

At this point, six months from the onset, she complained of finding the sessions burdensome and boring because he expected her to perform everyday for him just as her father did when she was a child. She had danced for him, drawn pictures for him, recited for him, and was never able to satisfy him. "He wanted me to be perfect, just as you want me to be a perfect patient. All I can do is to run away and try and live my own life. But no one will allow me to live my own life. Everyone wants to take a hand in it, especially you. I would like to get rid of them and you." At this point, the therapist was going on vacation, and the administrator asked the patient if she wanted an interim therapist. Her response was:

> I am content with Dr. Anthony. He's not perfect, but I like him. He is understanding and flexible, and we can even talk about movies. He will not go walking with me as some therapists do, but I am trying to change that. I told him not to interpret; that is his only fault. I need a good friend, and, if he wasn't being paid for doing all of this, he could be my friend. However, he shouldn't try to analyze me. Otherwise, I find him amiable.

A fragile therapeutic alliance had developed almost unnoticeably, and the question in the therapist's mind was: What lay behind this amiability? At about this time, a "twinship" developed between the patient and another adolescent girl also in the study, seeming to detract a lot of zest from the treatment situation, occasioning in the therapist a noticeable amount of counternarcissistic chagrin, called to his attention by the workgroup. The patient felt a strong sense of "merging" with this "twin," with whom she felt in communion because the girl was so much like her and understood her in a way the therapist did not. The mirroring with this alter ego took precedence over the idealizing process that had been slowly developing in the treatment. There was no question that more energy was attached to the "chumship," and the therapist had to wait for the few crumbs of cathexis that fell from the selfobject fiesta. In one session, she commented on his being colder since his return from vacation, speculated on the possibility of perhaps "a teensy-weensy bit of jealousy," and refused to answer when he asked her what came into her mind about this.

The twinship faded gradually and predictably, and she began to pay much more attention again to the therapist, chiefly in the direction of wanting to change him to her own image and likeness, of which she was quite aware. She first went through his wardrobe in theory, discarding some items of clothing and suggesting others that were better or suited him better or suited her better. She also went through the standard office equipment in his room and suggested fittings and furnishings that were "more real and less plastic." "I want you to be like I want you to be; then perhaps I could like you better." We were drawing to the end of the first year of treatment, and the workgroup stressed the narcissistic nature of the transference and cautioned the therapist not to set too much store on its strength. It was not unlikely that it might vanish overnight and leave the therapist disconsolately in the lurch. But they warmly toasted the year's work.

THERAPEUTIC TRANSFORMATIONS AT WORK

In the second year, some meaningful transformations began to take place. The acting out, whenever narcissistic hurt was experienced both in and outside therapy, lessened to a noticeable degree (as reported by the administrative staff), and sadness, often touching in its poignancy, made an unexpected appearance when least expected and was often accompanied by tears. The therapist felt less used, taken up, discarded, and not so much of a transitional object that could be taken up or put down as the mood of the moment took hold of her. The grist of the matter was that she now always came on time and never missed a session. She appeared also to be regarding him less as a part of herself and more of a person with a life of his own who continued to exist even when she was not there. In fact, she began writing him little notes from the cottage. The hateful devaluation of her parents was also beginning to diminish, as was evident in her family therapy. In fact, there seemed to be more object libido floating around and the suggestion of an oedipal awakening, although she fiercely denied that she ever had an "oedipal" interest in her father. She said, "If you believe this, we might as well give up this treatment because it's not going to go anywhere. Just stick to you and me, and it will be much more helpful." However, she went on to say that, when she was 6 years old, she fell in love with a playmate's daddy and would have liked to have lived in his house with him and her pal. "He was everything I would have wanted my father to have been. He was not so wrapped up in himself and his own thoughts. He could play with his daughter just as you probably played with your daughter—that is, if you had one.

She was not only doing well at the Lodge School but was regarded as a star pupil; one of the educators even considered sending samples of her poetry to a publisher for consideration—all of which stimulated ideas in the workgroup about Lou Andreas–Salome's thesis (1964) of creative narcissism, which she brought to Freud's attention (Anthony, 1998). There was now more reciprocity in the therapeutic situation, and she would bring poems in the making to the therapist without the fear that he would destroy them through analysis; in fact, she was more attuned to the helpfulness emanating from the therapeutic process and felt that the sharing of poetical imagery, in a free manner on both sides, sparked off, in her words, "childhood visions" that she tried also to transform into "insightful poetry," which was how she termed the new efforts. Most surprisingly for one who had so strenuously eschewed the patient role, she would lie on the couch from time to time, manifestly to help with versifying but often resorting to memory work with reminiscences both from early life but also from the early days of her treatment.

She began to talk about when and why things began to go wrong with her in her childhood but would also reconsider how and why things began to go wrong in the early days of her treatment and how at first she had hated the therapist because he was "so supercilious, arrogant, and Mr. Know-All who could cure her of everything under the sun, even her addiction to writing poetry." In the next period of treatment, it seemed to her that, like her parents, he wanted to make her more like her younger sister, who had always done everything just right and in the way that her parents desired. "She was the good daughter, and I was the bad daughter. You must think you are Pygmalion turning people into what you think is right. What about someone like me, who thinks that bad is good and that good is boring?"

On one occasion, she saw a letter on my desk (often a focus for her curiosity), addressed to "Sir James," which had been sent by a teasing colleague, and at once concluded that I had been knighted by the Queen at Buckingham Palace and that she was fortunate to be treated by such an eminent doctor (all this in a mocking but affectionate tone)! The therapist reported this to the workgroup, admitting that his narcissism had been stimulated and that he had been in no hurry to correct the patient's misconception. It was a joke, and both patient and therapist recognized it as such, to be enjoyed but not analyzed. The patient, however, continued, remarking that she understood that good doctors in England could also become lords. Perhaps their patients were also elevated and became honorables!

From the grapevine that was very active at Chestnut Lodge, she picked up the rumor that I had adopted a puppy (true), and she was immediately eager to see it. "It means that you are still adding to your family. I would also like a little baby puppy to cuddle and look after. I'm sure it would love me in return. I could take photos of the two puppies, and we could start a family album together. Just think of all the images you would get!" she added teasingly. The therapist said that he was glad to hear that she thought it took two to love, and she immediately replied that she had tried one-sided loving and that it was no good, no good at all. She had turned the corner about that, and, when he repeated "turned the corner," she at once flared up. "Whenever you echo me like that, it makes me feel very doubtful and uncomfortable. I have to reconsider it. It no longer seems to come from me but from you, as if you put something into my head." The therapist agreed that they had to be very clear about what came out of him and what came out of her because they were two very different people with their own minds and their own thoughts, and this seemed to relieve her.

On a later occasion, she reported that she had watched the video movie *Amadeus* and asked if the therapist would like her to bring it to a session so that they could watch it together (she had enjoyed it very much and felt that he would also). "Not much sadism!" He asked her what she had in mind about this particular movie and whether it would be of help to reveal something about the work they were doing together and something about themselves as therapist and patient. Unlike her reactions early in the treatment, she raised no objection to being dubbed a patient but answered seriously that, when she last watched it (the night before), she had identified herself as Salieri, who had talent but would never amount to anything, at least not anything grand. But, in thinking of herself as Salieri, she could only conclude that, in our setup, the therapist must be Amadeus. He found himself cautious in his response but then said lightheartedly that his new role was even more exalted than "Sir James" or even "Lord Anthony of Chestnut Lodge." Her next idealization could only be God or perhaps some role approaching that of her father in the media. (At the meeting of the workgroup, its members pointed out that, although patient and therapist were involved in grandiose play, the therapist was clearly uneasy with the situation and the counternarcissistic pressures thrust upon him.) The patient declared quite realistically that her father's achievement was no big deal as she thought about him now. When she was little, she had imagined his voice coming miraculously from the sky, but it was a very long time since she had listened to him. "I imagine I must have been suffering from a God complex then. Now I regard him more as a devil in a pathetic human form."

She then wanted to mention something that had happened at school that morning and that had made her very proud of herself, "but in a nice way." The teacher had given her a cutting from his plant, and she had potted it in a glass container that had made it look, everyone agreed, very beautiful—and she had done it all by herself. The therapist observed that the teacher had given her something that she had transformed into a thing of beauty, in the same way Mozart had given Salieri something that had made him feel much better about himself, even though he might continue to feel envious of Mozart's musical genius. The patient looked at him disdainfully and said that he was certainly not perfect and probably made as many mistakes in his everyday work as she did. She continued, "It's not that I dislike you, because I have really grown to like you, but you should stop analyzing everything. Why don't you just sit back for a change, take things for granted, and enjoy life. Stop analyzing life and just live it. You'll feel much better if you do." The workgroup applauded this as a nice piece of patient therapy and commented that Ferenczi (1955), the Hungarian analyst who believed in quid pro quo and was led to accord patients equal rights, would have enjoyed this interchange.

The next day, she came and showed the therapist a new unfinished poem, inviting his advice on what would make it perfect. She said that it did not feel perfect, and he wondered why she needed it to be perfect. As she well knew from her own experience, the world was not a perfect place, parents were not perfect, and certainly therapists were not perfect and did not and should not expect their patients to be perfect. Why could she not sit back and enjoy life. (Here she smiled.) Besides, he went on, he was not sure he would want to coauthor a poem with her, if it had to be absolutely perfect. She might be setting a trap for him, forcing him to become like her parents, who in the past had pushed her toward perfectionism. She heard him out but immediately complained that he was exaggerating the situation and, in fact, claiming too much credit. All she wanted was a little advice, not a copartnership.

That came from his own head. She wondered if he was not narcissistic, as they had called her in the psychologist's report. She then asked the therapist to read her poem aloud, which he did. Could he tell her whether it was good or bad? At this, the therapist demurred, stating that he was not an English teacher like her father or a poet like her mother, but said that he liked her poem because it had clearly come from inside her, that they had worked on it together with regard to the imagery, and that it had pleased them both in its present state. He did not know whether it was perfect, but he did not care if it was. They had played with words and images until the poem pleased them both, and he was happy to have been helpful to her in the important poetical aspect of her life. She remained unsatisfied but not angry.

At the next session, he asked her what she thought about their relationship after the previous day's disagreement. She at once became aloof and replied that there was no relationship that she knew of. He was paid by the hospital to see that she remained medically sound, and so he did his job. She hoped he was paid enough for his services; if not, she would speak to her father about it. She did not want him to be shortchanged. He then asked her, as she was doing well at school, whether she felt she could go home. She had an immediate angry outburst, "You surely are a very sensitive little doctor! Are you trying to get rid of me as my parents did when things did not quite go their way? I expect I've overstayed my welcome in this office," and flounced off. The workgroup members were upset and somewhat alarmed at what they correctly saw as the therapist's countertransferential aggressiveness, and they strongly encouraged him to make his peace with his young patient, as sending her home at this point might lead to a dangerous bit of acting out.

She came in disconsolately to the next session and decided to lie on the couch because she was tired, especially tired of him, and had not slept well in the night. He sat down and said he was glad to see her. There was a silence for about five minutes during which she sighed occasionally. She then began to talk slowly and softly without interruption from him:

I so like lying down in here. I don't think I've ever told you that. It feels so nice and warm. I'm thinking that, if someone was up there looking down on me lying here with my eyes closed, what would he be thinking?" She paused, and the therapist said quietly that He would not be looking down on her only but "on both of us together." He wondered what He would be thinking about that. There was another long silence, and then she said, "I do this at night before falling asleep. I imagine I'm talking to someone, and I start to remember things when I was very small. I feel small." Then she was silent again, and the therapist asked, "Who was someone?" She shook her head and then answered, "Who knows. Just someone. Could be anyone. It's all in the dark. Could be my father? You? Although I never think about you when I'm not here." She moved restlessly and began to gag. "Oh, god! There's something rotten inside me. Phlegm. I need to cough it up." She did but lay down again. The therapist asked, "Are there also good things that you need to keep inside?" She sounded mystified. "I don't know what you mean. There's nothing but phlegm inside my lungs from too much smoking. Are you thinking of food in my stomach? Because that's not good after it's been inside for hours. [pause] I know I'm exasperating you, but I can't think of anything good inside me. I'm so fucked up, nothing good would stay good inside me. Everything ends up becoming rotten. I'm a changing machine. Everything good is turned into bad." She closed her eyes again. "With my eyes closed, I don't have to keep thinking of you watching my every move and everything I say. [pause] I think of the sky arching over me, I mean us." And she giggled. "Mostly you're a do-do-head, but sometimes you say things that are true. I was lying in my bed last night and thinking all my weird thoughts, and I heard the staff talking, and I felt sure they were talking about me. Almighty me! Miss Paranoia! And I thought there are other people in the world beside me. Miss Superwoman! [silence] You would have been proud of me, or yourself. I must be changing. I don't think like I used to. My father thinks he knows everything I'm thinking. He's so almighty! I suppose you do too, Lord Anthony! Why do you both want to turn my thoughts into your thoughts? Do you possess me? Do I belong to you? Are you Superman? I used to think of you as just a nice guy, but, when I come here now, I get real scared no matter how calm I am before. I don't want to be dependent on anyone. I don't want to be straightjacketed by anyone. I just want to be my own person. [silence] Do you see any change in me?" The therapist hesitated before answering, and then he said, somewhat cautiously, that he experienced her now, compared with long before, as not talking at him but talking to him, as a person, and she flared up. "So I was a stinking, self-centered slob, and you changed me into my sister with a wave of your magic wand. But if I can change, so can you. I want you to take a walk with me." [The hospital grounds on a nice day can be quite idyllic] She continued, "You can call it walking therapy if you feel ashamed of doing something so unconventional. I'll lead, and you can just follow along." When the therapist expressed doubt, she got up and left, saying, "I'm very disappointed in you. I thought you were doing quite well. But you're afraid to change your ways, just like my parents. You could have written a paper on it!"

The next day, she came in highly elated. "Oh, Dr. A! I'm so happy and excited. Love is pouring down on me from all over. I feel so generous that I must share the wonderful thing with you." Her best friend, from whom she had been estranged, had written a reconciling note, and her current boyfriend, whom, to his embarrassment, she had been ardently pursuing, had penned a love poem to her; this was a patient struggling with gender problems! The therapist expressed his pleasure, remarking that it must feel good to find out how lovable she was. She admitted that she used to be convinced that no one loved her but herself. "What about your parents?" he asked. "Oh, them! But they belong to the past. I've done with them. I don't wish them any harm as I used to. But I'm so full of love today that I could even love them and even you, perhaps a very little bit."

The workgroup members were reassuring about the whole episode and its outcome, but they censured the therapist's "interruptive style" during her "free associations" on the couch, and they worried about his technical rigidities when dealing with an adolescent on the threshold of change. The therapist then told them that he was conscious of the narcissistic resistances behind her "bubbliness" and her "histrionic" passion. He saw the episode as more of a performance and was struck by her reference to his feeling "ashamed" about the walking therapy. He admitted that he would have been embarrassed trailing behind her on the hospital grounds with the staff wondering about the model therapist! What had struck him at the time was her complete absence of shameful affect, and he was reminded of her in grade school divesting herself of her dress in the classroom to show her pretty underwear. The absence of shame was like a hole in her personality. It also reminded him of what her father had once said about her—that she had never cared in the slightest what others thought about her, which was so unlike her sister, who was "normally shy." The workgroup members commented on his suggestibility, as in recent months they had turned to the exploration of that "Cinderella of unpleasant affects," so often overlooked and generally neglected. Was it making him overconscious and oversensitive to morbidity? The father had insisted that she had never manifested the least embarrassment in their Rousseau-like household about sphincter training, nudity, or "correct" social behavior. They had simply wanted her to grow as a "child of nature." But, if shame was missing, so apparently was guilt to a significant extent, and the workgroup began thinking in terms of sociopathy. Was she simply an abnormal product of a very abnormal household and a very abnormal child-rearing experience without overt guilt or shame-provoking mechanisms at work? But, the family was not isolated from its culture and its parochial effects, and certainly the parents in clinical discourse gave evidence of ego-ideal and superego systems. And how could he account for the family's excellent reputation in the community or the existence of a very proper younger sister who was a model student in the same school that her sister had attended and was a joy to her proud parents? Had these same proud parents learned some bitter lesson after the experience with the first child leading to an alteration of their ways? But, the parents still professed a strong belief in their Rousseau philosophy and were more inclined to consider some mysterious inborn error associated with bipolar neuropathology. There was certainly no obvious evidence of guilt absorbing shame in the developmental sequence (Erikson, 1950), and it was equally difficult to account for her relentless pursuit of perfection without some interplay of a guilt–shame cycle (Jacobson, 1964). It could be that her apparent shamelessness contained a good deal of countershame bravado in response to teasing by her peers—by the boys, especially, because of her frequent derogatory references to their "ridiculous little organs—certainly nothing to make a fuss about!"

In a still later session, the therapist told her that there had been a complaint from the cottage that she continued to spend hour-long sessions in the bathroom in the dark. The staff still suspected masturbation and felt that it should be taken up in her therapy, as it was proving quite a nuisance in everyday life. It was clearly not due to any minute examination for blemishes. "That's where I think," she responded. The therapist said to her that it might be more convenient for all concerned if she did her thinking as part of their mutual work together. She looked at him with some amazement, and, for the first time in their experience, she blushed profusely and dropped her eyes. Here, he thought, was shame, however admixed with guilt. After a significant pause, she said (still somewhat flushed and flustered), "I just couldn't do that here. You would analyze it and ruin it."

Shortly after, to the therapist's disappointment and chagrin, she was discharged from hospital and started attending a junior college.

Discussion

There have probably been many efforts, published and unpublished, to apply Rousseau's fantasied notions regarding the simplification of natural life as expressed in the famous *Dialogues* (1780), in which communicating ardently with nature led inevitably to peace and healing. Unfortunately, Rousseau himself was mentally unbalanced and strikingly narcissistic (one of his plays was entitled "Narcissism"), so that, taken lock, stock, and barrel rather than selecting judiciously from the wide range of wisdom that he offered might well contribute to the unbalancing of susceptible individuals, particularly if they treated it as a biblical text and followed it to the letter.

Furthermore, if there is a heavy genetic overloading, as in this case, the vulnerability to peculiar environmental mishandling might well result in unaccountable and paradoxical enhancements or breakdowns—transiently, recurrently, or permanently, depending on the therapeutic cooperation obtained. (In this case, the individual was violently opposed to any chemical interventions.)

Carrying out a psychotherapeutic treatment with an eye on both theory and technique (Freud's habitual mode of approach) can carry a backlash of counternarcissism that is not difficult for the astute patient to diagnose and even maliciously exploit. Adding a supervising workgroup to the picture brings further detriments into the already complex field. Attempts at theory seeking (or technique seeking) tend to summate the narcissisms of therapist and patient. In this context, one is reminded of Freud's terminating the analysis of Helene Deutsch because she had just an ordinary neurosis, and he could not find an hour for the famous Wolf Man!

The workgroup members, as they became more proficient and confident, also became more daring in their management of a senior colleague and gradually took on the dimensions of a Bion therapeutic group (Bion, 1959), gradually developing a more regressive atmosphere charged with transference and countertransference and projective identifications that influenced the therapist more than he liked or admitted to himself. At the work level, the group occupied itself with literature surveys, theoretical speculations, and the sharing of clinical vignettes; at the next level, there were personal disclosures of home and professional disclosures concerning cases that had not gone well and in which group criticism was sharp and could generate a good deal of heated altercation. At the level of "basic assumptions," there were dreams of the therapist falling ill and dying, resentment at any clinical dependence on him, and the uprising of oppositional leaders with their own messianic beliefs in our "extraordinary mission so often dismissed as the 'narcissism seminars.' " But, we have been doing what Freud would have recommended us to do, taking his own cue from Charcot—that is, continuing to look at phenomena as long as possible until "they seemed to tell the story by themselves," always, however, holding in mind that none of us were Charcots!

REFERENCES

Andreas-Salome, L. (1964), *The Freud Journal*, trans. & ed. S. A. Leavy. New York: Basic Books.

Anthony, E. J. (1973), Omnipotence and egocentrism during the impossible years. *Australian & New Zealand J. Psychiat.*, 7:227–232.

———— (1975), The influence of a manic–depressive environment on the developing child. In *Depression and Human Existence*, ed. E. J. Anthony & T. Benedek. Boston: Little Brown, pp. 279–315.

———— (1990), The long-term patient. *Adoles. Psychiat.*, 17:99–108. Chicago: University of Chicago Press.

———— (1998), Adolescent narcissism and adolescent narcissism-without-Narcissus: From adolescent fantasy to adult theory. In: *The Vulnerable Child*, ed. T. Cohen, M. Etezady & B. Pacella. New York: International Universities Press, pp. 1–28.

Bion, W. R. (1959), *Working in Groups*. New York: Basic Books.

Cohen, M. B. et al. (1954), An intensive study of twelve cases of manic–depressive psychosis. *Psychiat.*, 17:103.

Erikson, E. (1950), *Childhood and Society*. New York: Norton.

Ferenczi, S. (1932), Confusion of tongues between the adult and the child. *Inter. J. Psychoanal.*, 30:225–230.

———— (1955), *Final Contributions to the Problems and Methods of Psychoanalysis*. London: Maresfield Reprints.

Freud, A. (1969), Adolescence as a developmental disturbance. In: *The Writings of Anna Freud*, 7:39–47. New York: International Universities Press.

Freud, S. (1914), On narcissism: An introduction. *Standard Edition*, 14:73–102. London: Hogarth Press, 1957.

Green, A. (1983), *Narcissisme de Vie Narcissisme de Mort*. Paris: Editions de Minuit.

Grunberger, B. (1971), *Le Narcissisme*. Paris: Payot.

Inhelder, B. & Piaget, J. (1958), *The Growth of Logical Thinking from Childhood to Adolescence*. New York: Basic Books.

Jacobson, E. (1964), *The Self and the Object World*. New York: International Universities Press.

Katan, A. (1951), The role of "displacement" in agoraphobia. *Internat. J. Psycho-Anal.*, 32:41–50.

Kernberg, O. (1975), *Borderline Conditions and Pathological Narcissism*. New York: Aronson.

Kohut, H. (1971), *The Analysis of the Self*. New York: International Universities Press.

Mahler, M. S. & McDevitt, J. (1982), Thoughts on the emergence of the sense of self. *J. Amer. Psychoanal. Assn.*, 30:827–848.

Pulver, S. (1971), Can affects be unconscious? *Internat. J. Psycho-Anal.*, 52:347–354.

Pumpian-Mindlin, E. (1969), Vicissitudes of infantile omnipotence. *The Psychoanalytic Study of the Child*, 24:213. New Haven, CT: Yale University Press.

Rousseau, J. (1780), Dialogues. In: *Jean-Jacques Rousseau*, ed. L. G. Crocker. New York: Macmillan, 1968.

Winnicott, D. (1971), *Playing and Reality*. London: Tavistock.

Discussion

HOWARD D. LERNER

It is an honor to discuss Dr. Anthony's thought-provoking chapter on the treatment of the narcissistically disordered adolescent.

Psychoanalytic hospitals and residential treatment centers such as Chestnut Lodge are not only laboratories, so to speak, for the unfolding of rich dynamics, transference–countertransference enactments, and fascinating clinical research, but they also constitute their own unique society and culture that is passed down, almost mythically, and kept alive by staff discussion of past and present patients, by "special" patients that are thought of as "culture carriers," and by the presence of renowned senior clinicians. An important yet subtle aspect of Anthony's paper is the context—that is, the unique clinical setting of the Lodge and the role of a senior clinician, not only for the staff but also the patients. The patient's omnipotence and specialness were not only determined the day she was born but also began the first day she was admitted to the hospital, when Anthony chose to treat her.

In what follows, I review Anthony's paper, comment and elaborate on certain points, raise questions, and attempt to flesh out what appears to me to be significant theoretical and clinical issues. One can conceptualize the hospital treatment of disturbed adolescents in the following way. Upon admission, patients are given a certain amount of credit, which can be thought of as being deposited at the nursing station. When patients respond well to treatment, make few demands, in turn make the staff feel good about themselves, and, above all, do not act out along the lines of the three "no's"—sex, drugs, and aggression—they receive credit, which moves them more swiftly and safely toward discharge to a less restrictive and invasive environment. On the other hand, when patients act out and wreak havoc, there is often an initially subtle and subsequently not so subtle movement within the hospital community to extrude the patient. Initially, buzzwords such as *state hospital, medication,* and *Are we really sure of the diagnosis?* creep into staff discussion of patients and only vaguely conceal the wish to extrude. This is often a signal of incipient staff splits and the initiation of more intrusive, invasive treatment modalities such as seclusion, higher doses of medication, electroconvulsive therapy, and, eventually, transfer to a more restrictive, invasive environment such as a state hospital or a juvenile detention center. These remarks are offered with a view toward putting Anthony's paper in a particular context—that is, a psychiatric hospital setting that provides a fertile ground for countertransference both in its more narrow, restricting, hindering dimensions and in its broader, more information-providing functions. The hospital setting is a lively laboratory for enactments as pathways for communication within the treatment team, between staff and patients, and most intimately in the treatment situation between patients and therapists. Enactments express what is not yet verbalized. They are conduits of memories, hidden resistances, and fantasies waiting to happen; they are signals of what to anticipate and previews of coming attractions; they are invaluable guides in our effort to explore and come to better understand the subtle and pervasive interaction between patient and therapist that form the core of the treatment process. In a human relationship, the study of one individual, no matter which one, is likely to illuminate the behavior of the other.

In his introductory remarks, Anthony's description of the study group, the pitfalls of working with the narcissistic adolescent patient, and his role as therapist–patient matchmaker immediately recalls a classic paper ("The Ailment") by another Englishman, Thomas Main (1953). Main's paper reflects what can be learned from difficult patients and one's own countertransference to them. Anthony's preamble quotes Freud as saying, "Narcissism is a borderline concept that should not be used as a key to everything." I wonder if Freud misjudged the significance of the contribution that he made to the study of narcissism. His original paper, "On Narcissism" (1914), and his refinement of it have had a major impact on psychoanalysis (e.g., our understanding of relationships). The role of multiple theories of narcissism, which Anthony touched upon, raises the interesting question of the relationship between theory and treatment and how sometimes theory can provide an indispensable guiding function, whereas at other times it can be an interference and obstacle.

Anthony's chilling description of the manic–depressive milieu of the patient's family and the parents' own sense of having had "appalling parental models" reminds one of Shengold's (1991) sensitive description of "soul murder"—the effects of trauma suffered by children at the hands of deranged, cruel, and unfeeling adults. The patient's parents, by virtue of their chronic and fixed defensive reactions to overstimulating experiences, were deprived of the capacity for love, for feeling joy, and indeed for feeling any sustained intensity of positive emotion. Their fantasies, conscious and unconscious, were drenched with sadomasochism and rage. For example, when the patient was born, the mother said:

> We knew from the start that we had a wonderful gifted child who had unique ways of looking at the world and would follow her own drummer towards her creative goals. We are prepared to

give her all the latitude she needed in order to achieve these, and the best home and learning environment possible. *Our* goal was to see her go out into life with her spirit and talents intact.

Their noble attempt to create a utopian universe for their child, free from any frustration, limitation, or pain, was the parents' way of externalizing their own omnipotent fantasies onto their child and had absolutely nothing to do with their daughter's realistic abilities or reality. The gap between the parents' expectations, ambitions, and fantasies, on the one hand, and the child's real capacities and talents, on the other hand, is truly the "dilemma of the gifted child." The patient can be thought of as the daughter of soul-murdered parents who, because of weakness of character and inability, were unable to be "good enough" parents. These parents were chronically anxious and terrified of their own anger, which paradoxically created an almost pure culture of sadomasochism.

One is struck by Anthony's description of his patient's development, including her fearless risk-taking and absence of separation anxiety, her own language and private speech, her steadfast refusal to acquiesce to norms, her hostile insistence on not being interrupted, and her incoherent, disorganized world, which included such raucous behavior as taking her dress off in class as an action that could actually manipulate her teachers into praise. These descriptions were quite consistent with the formulations of Jack and Kerry Novick (1991) in their paper, "Some Comments on Masochism and the Delusions of Omnipotence from a Developmental Perspective." According to the Novicks, the child's real capacity to elicit the appropriate response from parents is the origin of feelings of competence, effectiveness, and reality-based positive self-esteem. In normative development, the capacity of the mother–infant couple to repair inevitable breaches in the empathic bond is an equally important source of feelings of competence and self-regard. A wide spectrum of positive feelings, from contentment to joy, becomes associated with competent interactions and comes to signify empathic interaction. According to Novick and Novick (1991), "pleasure is dependent and regulated by the capacity of each partner for realistic perception and interaction with the other, which leads in turn to the experience of having an actual effect on the other" (p. 312).

It appears that, from birth, the patient's capacity to elicit needed responses was ineffectual. Despite the omnipotent, utopian fantasies the parents externalized onto her, and as loving as their intentions may have been, they seriously sabotaged their daughter's confidence in her ability to evoke needed, reality-based responses and interactions. The real failure of the parents to achieve competent interactions with their daughter forced her to turn to a world of omnipotent solutions. Novick and Novick (1991) distinguished between fantasies that enhance the real capacities of the self, perhaps more akin to grandiosity, and those aimed at denying and transforming the pain and inadequacy of the parent–child relationship. Although the classical psychoanalytic view holds that it is the failure of omnipotence that forces the child to turn to reality, it is clear that, in the patient's development of her own language and roles, it was the failure of reality, in the form of "not good enough" parents, that forced her to turn to omnipotent solutions.

It is safe to assume that the early and consistent failure of the parents to meet their daughter's appropriate need for competent interactions— including the first psychic organizer of "no" and realistic limit setting and appropriate discipline, which emanates from it—created a feeling of intense, helpless rage in the toddler, which was defended against by omnipotent fantasies of control, rescue, and destructiveness. Drawing from Novick and Novick's (1991) formulation, one can assume that the normative narcissistic blows of oedipal exclusion, which forces the recognition of the real physical differences between the sexes as well as between child and adult, were experienced by the patient as yet another failure to evoke the wished-for response from objects and intensified all earlier failures, leaving her in a helpless, terrified rage. The birth of a sister at age 4, perhaps her first taste of knowledge of the real world, was experienced as an expulsion from Paradise and may have been experienced as her first brush with shame. It appears that the patient's latency period, rather than providing the opportunity for competent interactions in the real world, with pleasure experienced through real achievements, with controls internalized and infantile wishes sublimated, prompted her to retreat into omnipotent fantasies of control and manipulation of others in order to maintain self-esteem. The power to evoke positive responses from her teachers despite unconventional, hostile behavior, demonstrated how she could manipulate people into magically supporting her narcissism.

By adolescence, it became increasingly difficult for her to deny and distort reality without resorting to escalating self-destructive behavior to compensate for decaying omnipotent fantasies or extreme loneliness, withdrawal, and detachment. The adolescent experience of competence and pleasure in separate, gender-distinct adult behavior such as genital sexuality poses a tremendous threat to omnipotence. Pleasure, according to Novick and Novick (1991), leaves the adolescent feeling ordinary and not special. The patient's preoccupation and identification with Marilyn Monroe represented a particularly elegant compromise formation. No longer able to be the "creative butterfly" whose achievements were at once magical, effortless, and swift, she became increasingly impulsive and ruthless as her omnipotent fantasies became obviously and disturbingly alienated from reality. Although many would describe the "narcissistic adolescent" as a redundancy, the destructive omnipotence manifested by this patient and by many disturbed adolescents is not part of normal development; that is, the omnipotent fantasies arise in the context of sadomasochistic helplessness and become part of a line of deviant development that enlists rage to break all reality constraints at each and every phase of development (Novick & Novick, 1991). In normative adolescents, narcissism is more selective and is often accompanied by altruism and the appreciation of others.

Anthony's willingness to watch videos with his patients shows an important quality for therapists working with adolescents. Adolescents use a variety of modalities of communicating, and so we must be prepared to adapt to the ways in which they communicate. The patient's fantasy that Anthony was writing a book about her using the pseudonym of "Pandora Peterkin" (Peter Pan) is not only about the child who refused to grow up but is a story of a child's repair of injured narcissism in the light of a particular developmental conflict between the fear of adult sexuality and the fear of losing "the nursery." In essence, how can one safely grow up without suffering too much narcissistic damage? This phase of treatment also demonstrated how the patient would pathologically convert negative reactions to her outlandish clothing into signs of uniqueness and specialness. There was not only "something very young, naive, and innocent about all her attitudes and activities," but they were embellished with hostile omnipotence. The patient's exhibitionistic and defiant acting out (AWOL, drug taking, shoplifting) could be understood as a repetition and a putting into action of what was too painful to experience as feelings and expressed through words. The uproar she caused in the hospital and her own wondering whether the "next stop downward would be a state hospital" were subtle and not so subtle signs that she was running out of credit, that some among the staff wanted to get rid of her (not unlike her experience of her father and the birth of her sister), and that the hospital was all too dangerously and unconsciously taking part in an enactment with the patient by taking the shape of her family.

Her constant refrain, "I told him not to interpret . . . he shouldn't try to analyze me," speaks to the patient's subjective experience of her therapist's interpretive role. From her perspective, she experienced interpretations as intrusive and as taking something away from her, as blemishing her narcissism. We tend to emphasize how interpretation integrates and adds meaning to the patient's experience, but interpretation can also take fantasies and previous treasured meanings away. We must be particularly sensitive to this aspect of interpretation in dealing with patients who manifest hostile omnipotence as a defense against helplessness. With magical, omnipotent beliefs that they are both sexes or oedipal victors, that achievements come "quick and easy," without effort, and that there are no limits, interpretations can only be experienced initially as taking away—as intrusive, destructive, and dangerous.

The phases of treatment described by Anthony seem to revolve around an initial resistance to acknowledging and putting into words aggressive and libidinal drive derivatives for fear, among other things, that they would lead to the destruction of herself and important others. As the working alliance—that is, the positive transference—began to take hold in actions increasingly replaced by words, significant strides were made in the areas of self–other differentiation, including a greater tolerance for pleasure in her ego capacities as they became increasingly coordinated with reality. In fact, the dangers of pleasure in reality and its threat to the omnipotent system of controlling the actions and feelings of others, as well as denying reality constraints, hit home when Anthony commented on how "happy" he was to be "helpful to her." Here, a significant enactment took place in which Anthony greeted his patient's sudden aloofness and devaluation of the question "if she felt she could go home." As treatment progressed and indeed deepened, it appeared that the patient's delusion of omnipotent control as a response to helplessness, frustration, and rage, and its connection to their infantile roots, came increasingly into conflict with the reality principle of self-esteem based on competent interactions with her therapist and a greater acceptance of limitations, and a deeper involvement in the real world became evident. These changes were not only the result of a Winnicottian holding environment, reparenting, or empathy alone but a direct result of Anthony's well-timed, thoughtful interpretations and working through of what the patient experienced as a communicative mismatch.

One of the most fascinating aspects of Anthony's paper involves the concept of shamelessness. Shame is often thought of as a problem, and one wonders about its relation to guilt, but Anthony raises the important question: What about those who do not experience shame? One is reminded of Glenn Close's portrayal of Alex in the movie *Fatal Attraction* and the biographical cinema *Camille Claudel* and how the absence of shame omnipotently empowers the person to do whatever he or she wants to do, as if there were no reality constraints. Among other things, shame, like guilt, provides a certain inhibition. Shamelessness presupposes the absence of such inhibition. One can ask if the capacity for shame is a developmental achievement or an aberration. Although we can certainly take the concept of shame along classical drive lines in terms of issues of toilet training and disgust, one can also think of shame in terms of self-esteem and its relation to omnipotence with the patient's provocative, unconventional omnipotent behavior—a defense against the smallness of shame as well as helplessness. In terms of theory, if one can think of shamelessness as being an expression of omnipotence, then shame can be thought of as a signal affect leading to an omnipotent defense. The affect of shame occurs when individuals experience themselves as not living up to an ideal standard that they accept. Shame is related to "I cannot see myself as I want to see myself and be seen by others." Shamelessness assumes that perfectionistic ideals and goals are being met magically, the individual is embodying perfectionistic standards, and "I can have what I want, when I want it, the moment I want it, with 100% efficiency, or else!"

Shame in this sense can be conceptualized as the counterpart of signal anxiety, as a signal affect in cases of narcissism (Melvin Bornstein, personal communication, March 1993). Shame signals the danger of impending narcissistic mortification along the lines of omnipotence, control, self-esteem, and safety. Experientially, it has to do with self-exposure, the exposure of *me* and the sense of being out of control. Shame, leading to guilt, as a developmental achievement, presupposes self–other differentiation and the capacity to see oneself through the eyes of another—it demands the reality-based presence of another person.

In conclusion, I appreciate the opportunity to discuss Anthony's rich paper and would like to end with some of Rilke's poetic musing, which, I believe, captures the aim of treatment with narcissistically disturbed adolescents: "Once the realization is accepted even between the closest human beings, infinite distance continues to exist, a wonderful living side by side can grow up, if they succeed in loving the distance between them, which makes it possible for each to see the other whole against the sky" (Mood, 1975).

REFERENCES

Freud, S. (1914), On narcissism: An introduction. *Standard Edition*, 14:73–102. London: Hogarth Press, 1957.

Main, T. (1953), The ailment. *J. Brit. Psycholog. Society*, 19:129–145.

Mood, J. (1975), *Rilke on Love and Other Difficulties*. New York: Norton.

Novick, J. & Novick, K. (1991), Some comments on masochism and the delusions of omnipotence from a developmental perspective. *J. Amer. Psychoanal. Assn.*, 39:307–328.

Shengold, L. (1991), A variety of narcissistic pathology stemming from parental weakness. *Psychoanal. Quart.*, 60:86–89.

8   SNATCHING DEFEAT FROM THE JAWS OF SUCCESS: SELF-DESTRUCTIVE BEHAVIOR AS AN EXPRESSION OF AUTONOMY IN YOUNG WOMEN

ELIZABETH PERL

Risky and even self-destructive behavior is strikingly prevalent in clinical work with adolescent girls and young adult women. Such behavior can certainly be frightening to the therapist, who may be tempted to take on the job of reigning in this dangerous acting out by attempting to manage whatever appears to be overwhelming to the adolescent. This clinical stance reflects the notion that self-destructive behavior may represent evidence of entrenched psychopathology and impairment in the capacity to cope with feelings and impulses. In this essay, I suggest that much of this self-destructive behavior may be part of the normative, highly conflicted struggle among young women to separate from long and close bonds with family, especially mother. By hurting or defeating herself, the adolescent can rebel and assert her power without actually carving out a viable niche for herself in the world that could take her away from emotional or practical dependence. Given this developmental function, high-risk behavior need not be regarded solely as a manifestation of regression or as a permanent or fixed adaptation, but rather it may be part of an evolving struggle with autonomy that includes progressive strivings. I am not suggesting that all adolescent risk-taking is necessarily self-destructive or self-defeating in nature, and I am not suggesting that any such sort of destructive behavior merely be accepted as healthy or adaptive for young women. Rather, I argue that, even when risk taking is mostly self-destructive, there may be an underlying progressive developmental struggle taking place in relationship to a caregiver, which may include the parent, the therapist, or both. Given the developmental function of such risk taking, the therapeutic effort to control these symptoms may have a paradoxical effect, fueling the drive to defy parental/therapeutic authority through self-destruction. The provocative or dangerous aspects of the adolescent's behavior here may function to disguise from the therapist, and from the adolescent herself, the self-assertive nature of this emotional and interpersonal struggle.

If a therapist becomes caught up in the regressive, pathological aspects of self-destructive behavior, he or she may overlook misguided autonomous strivings. Any attempt on the therapist's part to control the self-destructive aspects of the adolescent's behavior may collude with a denial of the patient's separateness, particularly the developmental mandate for independent decision-making. The stage is then set for the adolescent or young adult to assert her autonomy by overwhelming the therapist's protective efforts, persisting with self-destructive behaviors in the face of well-intentioned interpretation and limit setting. Both the adolescent's own fears of being hurt or defeated in efforts toward independence, and her ambivalence surrounding autonomy, may be denied when the therapist assumes responsibility for the adolescent's behavior. A split can be created where the adolescent embraces only the thrill of risk, safe in the knowledge that her therapist will take on any disavowed feelings, particularly her fears and wishes for protection. The patient's inner conflict may then be played out interpersonally, as power struggles with the therapist come to dominate the treatment, shifting the focus from exploration of the adolescent's own ambivalence regarding her choices.

Conflict surrounding the prospect of increased independence may emerge most dramatically at transition points, which often become times of heightened risk. Self-destructive or self-defeating behavior at these critical junctures can sabotage the opportunity for genuine autonomy. Snatching defeat from the jaws of success, the adolescent systematically spoils opportunities to realize profit from her achievements, giving in to destructive inclinations just at the moment she might have been able to seize something different and better. For example, in psychotherapy, self-destructive acting out often erupts at pivotal points, when the therapist is most hopeful about the possibility for departure from problematic emotional, familial, and social patterns. Any step forward—such as graduation, a first job, a new loving romantic relationship, or movement toward a stable, independent living situation—may be associated with the risk of self-destructive repercussions.

The following examples illustrate both passive and active forms of such self-sabotage. A very beautiful young woman, eager to please and guided by loyalty to family and friends, remains committed to a dead-end relationship with a boyfriend who is possessive and erratic and who has explicitly stated his unwillingness to commit to her. She is passively embracing a path that is self-defeating, given that she deeply wants a long-term, committed romantic partner. In the process, she is ensuring that her primary attachment will remain securely with her parents. Another young woman, whose sexual relationships had previously been limited to men who are abusive or demeaning, becomes steadily involved with a new boyfriend who treats her with genuine affection and respect. She then actively impulsively seduces her new boyfriend's roommate and engages him in intercourse, thereby destroying any possibility of a continued healthy involvement with her boyfriend.

The disturbing, often frightening nature of such risk and damage, especially when it comes on the heels of an opportunity for something better, tends to elicit a pull to exert some control over the adolescent. The inclination on the part of the therapist to try to rescue, and fight to preserve the patient's progress, colludes with the adolescent's wish to maintain a sense that she has the power to avoid possible failure, rejection, loss, and narcissistic injury. The therapist who assumes the role of protector may encounter angry resistance, including protests that the therapist cannot ensure the patient's emotional or physical safety. This, of course, is true, not only because the therapist cannot control the adolescent, but because he or she cannot control the adolescent's world. In the process of attempting to safeguard the adolescent, the therapist may be drawn into a hostile–dependent struggle that gratifies the regressive wish to be tangling with a caregiver rather than facing emotional and interpersonal risks in the world of peer relationships.

The acting out seen in psychiatric settings, which can assume life-threatening proportions, may be an extreme version of the risk taking or other rebellious behavior associated with normative conflict around female separation-individuation. This essay employs a psychodynamic perspective in exploring both the developmental functions and the clinical implications of risk taking among young women. The discussion considers gender-related patterns in psychopathology, specifically the trend among adolescent females toward internalizing disorders, particularly depression, in which aggression is directed toward the self, in contrast to the externalizing conduct disorders characteristic of boys.

This tendency toward internalization among young women is explored within the context of familial and larger social influences that inhibit the opportunity to express aggression in the form of self-assertive and competitive strivings out in the world. Turning to the therapeutic relationship, I consider how the threat of self-destructive behavior can contribute to the development of a hostile–dependent bond between the adolescent and her therapist, in which the therapist takes responsibility for the patient in a manner that replicates some of the regressive, dependent aspects of the mother–daughter relationship. I also explore interventions that allow opportunity for direct expression of anger and self-interest within the therapeutic relationship, thus offering the adolescent an experience with separation and individuation that is fueled by self-assertion rather than self-destruction.

Adolescence as a Time of Heightened Emotional Conflict for Girls

Empirical findings suggest that, for females, relative to the childhood years, adolescence is associated with increased incidence of psychiatric difficulties. Almqvist (1986) summarizes these trends: "Before adolescence, girls are healthier and boys are less healthy. After adolescence this state of affairs is reversed. Even in early adolescence it is evident that the frequency of symptoms in girls is more nearly equal to that in boys at younger ages" (p. 295). These empirical studies suggest the presence of gender-linked patterns not only in the rate and onset of symptoms but in the nature of psychiatric difficulties reported among adolescents (Schonert-Reichl and Offer, 1992). Specifically, girls become vulnerable to internalizing disorders including depression, anxiety, somatization, and eating disorders (Kashani et al., 1987; Bernstein, Garfinkel, and Hoberman, 1989). Severe psychiatric disorder is equally common among boys and girls in adolescence, but females are more likely to be diagnosed as borderline and to seek treatment for depression and suicidal ideation (Almqvist, 1986). In contrast, problems of conduct disorder, hyperactivity, and aggression are more prevalent among males (Kashani et al., 1987), demonstrating continuity with the higher rate of behavior disorders reported for boys throughout childhood.

The increased incidence of internalizing pathology among girls suggests that, beginning in adolescence, aggression tends to be turned toward the self in the form of self-defeating or self-destructive behavior. This gender-linked pattern of psychiatric symptoms may reflect an associated inhibition in the capacity to acknowledge that particular events or interactions have made the girls feel hurt or angry. Even when they are able to overcome this reluctance and recognize the emotional impact of injurious events, young women may fail to let the other know how they were affected (e.g., to put their anger into words that can then be addressed in the interaction). This pattern may help to explain why adolescent women are at risk for anorexia (with the associated self-starvation and relentless exercise), bulimia and self-induced purging, attachment to abusive or exploitative partners, and self-mutilation, all of which represent different ways of treating the self harshly and aggressively. These behaviors may feel angry and aggressive to therapists, parents, or others who feel responsible for the adolescent, yet, here, self-destructive actions rather than specific verbal communications are used to express feelings. By hurting herself, the adolescent is inflicting something on the therapist, and this reliance on action avoids the process of acknowledging and verbalizing angry feelings in the context of a relationship. In addition, symptoms of depression, hopelessness, anxiety, low self-esteem, or self-deprecating attitudes often handicap efforts at competition and self-assertion. The upsurge in this type of emotional and social difficulty in adolescence suggests that conflict in managing and expressing aggression begins to disrupt female adjustment when pressures surrounding separation and autonomy intensify. In the discussion to follow, I explore some of the emotional, relational, and social influences that can subvert the young developing woman's capacity to integrate aggression with the pursuit of intimacy, self-interest, and achievement.

Rebellion as an Attempt Both to Achieve and to Sabotage Autonomy

Feminist writers have identified gender-related expectations that can interfere with the young woman's ability to deal productively with aggression. Miller (1991) suggests that anger and assertiveness are often pathologized or stigmatized for females, except when expressed on behalf of a dependent other: "Women are not supposed to use their own activity for their own self-initiated and self-defined goals or for their own development. From very early in life, women have been led to believe that their life activities should be for others and that their main task is to make and maintain relationships—relationships that serve others" (pp. 184–185). Given this orientation, adolescence may be particularly conflictual for young women because their primary developmental task is to extricate themselves from a caregiving bond that nurtures both the daughter and the mother. Aggression is an inherent part of this separation process because the daughter must reject some aspects of her mother's wish to nurture, and she must also reject her own wish for approval from mother in order to embrace an independent identity. Spezzano (1993) explains that "establishing oneself as a subject involves authorizing oneself to bring new meanings into the world and then carrying those meanings into the subjectivities of the mother and all the other potential authorities that follow her in one's life" (p. 104). Spezzano suggests that any separation is an act of "emotional violence to the symbolic mother, even if our intent is not to do violence but simply to act on our own interest, excitement, and enthusiasm" (p. 105).

Stone Center publications (Jordan et. al., 1991) have recognized the adaptive aspects of the female developmental trajectory, particularly the enhanced capacity for intimacy derived from the continuity of the mother–daughter bond. Such recognition of relational skills as a part of successful adjustment represents a step beyond the more narrow focus on power and achievement previously found in the literature. An effort is clearly being made to shift from a concern with separation and self-empowerment, emphasized in the study of male development, to an appreciation of the value of attachment and intimacy, as it is cultivated in the course of female development. The result is an identification of different lines of normative development associated with positive male and female adjustment.

However, by differentiating the indicators of adjustment for women and men to relational capacities versus achievement capacities, this feminist perspective may function to promote gender-based dichotomies, thus limiting our perceptions and understanding of women and men. I would further argue that this dichotomy fails to offer a more integrated understanding of how different expressions of power, intimacy, competition, and attachment transcend gender lines. The emphasis on gender differences leads us to think in terms of polarities, which is overly restrictive with regard to our expectations regarding the adjustment of men and women. For example, a focus on competition among men can result in a tendency to overlook expressions of nurturance.

Even in the midst of competition, male "adversaries" may experience feelings of mutual connection and support, and they may seek opportunities to challenge each other to perform better or to grow emotionally from the battle. In a similar vein, Kaftal (1991) suggests that "transference expressions of longing for intimate male relatedness may go unrecognized or misunderstood" in the treatment relationship (p. 321). For developing young women, it is more likely that inclinations toward self-assertion and competition may be overlooked or misinterpreted. This might include a failure to recognize the place of aggression and self-interest in caregiving relationships, as well as the importance of competitive relationships as part of a full social and working life.

This tendency toward dichotomy and polarity in our view of gender has been criticized by Goldner (1991) as an "obsession" among feminists. Goldner argues that "gender itself is pathogenic" (p. 270), explaining that "conventionalized gender assumptions dictate psychic terms that simultaneously require compliance and provoke resistance: men can never be 'needy,' women can never put themselves 'first' " (p. 267). Polarity in our notions of feminine and masculine can create conflict in personal identity (Dimen, 1991). It is ironic that the Stone Center writings, which were intended to reduce the conflicts between male-based expectations and norms and women's actual experiences, unwittingly created new identity conflicts by focusing on too narrow a range of experience for men and women (M. Pfeiffer, personal communication, 1995). Such a formulation does not capture the full complexity and range of our ways of being and relating. Horner (1991), for example, writes, "To the extent that [the girl's] aggression is tied to her identity with her father, she is likely to feel the conflict between her sense of being powerful or strong and her femininity" (p. 228).

Leadbeater, Blatt, and Quinlan (1995) oppose the inclination to shape expectations regarding male and female adjustment according to gender-based generalizations:

Research showing that women are more concerned with relationships and appearance should not be taken as inevitable, normative, or as the biologically-based attributes of women. In this case, *what is*, clearly is not *what ought to be*. The unfortunate trend of reinforcing stereotypical visions of women as self-disclosing, empathic, relational, and caring and of men as guarded, assertive, independent, separate, and rational serves to normalize, rather than challenge, gender differences that may create vulnerabilities to psychopathology [pp. 19–20].

Stereotyped notions of the woman as nurturer provide a context in which self-depriving behavior is not only normalized but even glorified. For example, aggression may be channeled into self-destructive or self-defeating action that is expressed by consistently deferring or declining fulfillment of one's own needs to attend to the needs of the other. In this light, angry self-sabotage may be represented as a form of self-sacrifice for another person. Such veiled expression of aggression may become acceptable, as it is more congruent with the stereotypic and socially acceptable female role. Within the context of caregiving, any underlying wish for power and control can thereby be disguised or denied.

Nurturance is central in both the girl's attachment to her mother and in gender-linked identification with mother. If a mother's job is to nurture, and a daughter's job is to be nurtured, the open expression of anger and aggression may be experienced by both mother and daughter as a threat to the caregiving bond. Adolescent rebellion may seem to jeopardize their relationship, and, out of this fear, the daughter may adopt an increasingly counterdependent or distant stance. The mother may feel that her daughter has withdrawn emotionally because their bond has been lost. Yet, in fact, the pressure to disengage and rebel is more intense when feelings of attachment are more powerful. Furthermore, the process of rebellion itself can be a test of the solidity of the bond: The adolescent is able to separate most effectively when she feels that mother will remain emotionally available and invested throughout this struggle. The mother–daughter relationship can be so close that interpersonal boundaries become blurred, further complicating attempts to understand adolescent rebellion. The adolescent may be trying to hurt herself by hurting her mother, or she may be trying to hurt her mother by hurting herself—or both dynamics could be in operation at the same time.

The discussion to follow explores these conflicting emotional, interpersonal, and developmental pressures within the context of a mother–daughter relationship. For a young woman, the primary conflict centers on the gender-specific struggle to integrate strivings for autonomy and power with this long-standing nurturing bond with her mother. Rebellion and separation may be experienced as a threat to their nurturing tie, to this aspect of mother's self-esteem and identity, and to the girl's own sense of femininity. Self-destructive behavior may act out both sides of the adolescent's struggle with autonomy and dependence: The daughter is defying her mother's role as caregiver while she is simultaneously demonstrating her desperate need for guidance and protection.

Interplay Between Attachment and Anger in Mother–Daughter Relationships

Girls are faced with the paradoxical task of attaching to and identifying with a mother from whom they must separate in adolescence (Chodorow, 1978; G. Friedman, 1980). This contrasts with the agenda for boys, who must separate from mother in the first years of life to establish a primary identification with father. "A son's male core gender identity develops away from his mother. The male's sense of self, as a result, becomes based on a more fixed 'me'– 'not me' distinction" (Chodorow, 1989, p.110). Although both male and female infants establish a differentiated sense of self in the first years of life, the girl's preoedipal attachment to mother is deeper and more prolonged. For boys, this shift away from attachment to mother in early childhood facilitates the task of separation later on in adolescence. The teenage boy has greater opportunity to launch into adulthood relatively unencumbered by ties and conflicts that could interfere with the wholehearted, aggressive pursuit of achievement.

By contrast, prolonged mother–daughter attachment can foster more conflict regarding the pursuit of independent ventures, as loyalties and childhood dependencies compete with the press to claim a separate place for one's self in the world. The exclusive nature of the tie with mother extends throughout childhood, allowing the "two person relationship of infancy" to remain primary (Chodorow, 1978, p. 96). Other familial and extrafamilial relationships supplement rather than supersede the primary bond with mother. Benjamin (1991) asserts that "girls' ambivalence around separation may be more intense than that of boys because of the bond of likeness between mother and daughter" (p. 285). Chodorow (1978) suggests that a mother's attitude toward her daughter is shaped by the mother's gender identification:

151

Because they are the same gender as their daughters and have been girls, mothers of daughters tend not to experience these infant daughters as separate from them in the same way as do mothers of infant sons. In both cases, a mother is likely to experience a sense of oneness and continuity with her infant. However, this sense is stronger, and lasts longer, vis-a-vis daughters. Primary identification and symbiosis with daughters tend to be stronger and cathexis of daughters is more likely to retain and emphasize narcissistic elements, that is to be based on experiencing a daughter as an extension or double of herself [p. 109].

An adolescent's assertion of differences from her mother can violate a long-standing unity that has been based, at least in part, on the experience of seeing or seeking one's self in the other. A daughter's ambivalence around separation may well be shared by her mother, with maternal nurturing serving both to support and to suppress her daughter's efforts to individuate. In fact, if mother were to stretch her loving tolerance to embrace the adolescent's aversive or risky rebellious behavior, this act of nurturance could undermine her daughter's efforts to achieve an independent identity that needs to be defined, in part, through opposition. Furthermore, the absence of parental anger or other emotional reaction could trigger an escalation of the rebellion that would be aimed at forcing the mother to acknowledge that her daughter is different and separate. To support individuation, the mother must somehow incorporate tempered aggression and opposition into her efforts to nurture.

For the adolescent, there is much at risk in the process of claiming an independent identity. A daughter may fear that, by rejecting her mother's guidance and nurturance, she will hurt or destroy her mother, damage their bond, provoke rejection, or otherwise jeopardize a relationship that seems closer than any she might be able to imagine. Consequently, the adolescent may seize upon self-defeating forms of rebellion as a means of denying her attachment and dependence, provoking rejection so as to fend off a sense of loss. In this defensive maneuver, the aggression inherent in the individuation process is embraced to excess, perhaps communicating that the tie to mother cannot be loosened without some violence being done to it. The adolescent may be grappling with the fear that she can only achieve autonomy at the expense of their bond.

ELIZABETH PERL

The Struggle with Aggression and Dependence
in the Therapeutic Relationship

The caregiving nature of the therapist's role allows for re-creation of the dynamics of the mother–daughter relationship, even to the extreme of producing a hostile–dependent stalemate. The clinical challenge at this point is to find ways not only to capture the experience of these unresolved conflicts between attachment and separation but also to create opportunity for a different outcome. Because group therapy introduces a forum for peer competition and support, it can provide an ideal setting in which to address separation-related issues. In the context of group, the adolescent's personal needs and attachment to the therapist must be balanced with the needs of other members and the opportunity to establish independent peer connections. This constellation of relationships affords the adolescent room to explore varying sides of her conflicts around providing and receiving nurturance, submitting and asserting power, and dealing with anger, competition, and aggression in close relationships.

To illustrate this process, I describe a clinical dilemma that arose in group with a young woman who entered treatment because of feelings of depression and hopelessness and a history of self-destructive behavior. One day several months into treatment, Vivian appeared for group looking obviously upset. However, she refused to make a bid for a turn to talk, even when encouraged to do so, stating that she did not want to "hog" time or burden others with her problems. She may have feared that she would feel rejected if she asked for time and encountered any resistance, or she may have felt hurt that no one simply insisted that she work. I felt concerned about her distress, but I was also irritated by her refusal to use words to ask for help. Through her passivity, she was shifting some of the burden of responsibility for her needs to me, the group leader. In order to attend to her distress, I could have tried talking her into taking a turn, or I could have simply assigned her a turn and let her use her time as she wished. Either option would have required breaking with group procedures, as it was expected that each member would take responsibility for asking for time to talk on a given day. I was reluctant to indulge what I perceived as a regressive play for special treatment, which then might compound the gratification and power associated with her passive position. At the same time, I knew that my choice to operate as usual could be taken as rejection or neglect and that she might respond with more dramatic acting out.

Although I was concerned about what Vivian would do after the group ended, I felt that, over the long haul, it would be more dangerous for Vivian and other group members if this type of acting out was allowed to overturn the limits of the group. Any adolescent from an emotionally unresponsive family background might be tempted at times to passively force others to respond to her needs through the threat of self-destructive behavior. In his work with suicidal patients, Hendin (1981) described this type of dynamic in the treatment relationship as a form of coercive bondage in which the patient attempts to manipulate the therapist with threats of death. In further exploration of the clinical implications of coercive bondage, Maltsberger (1994) considered the dangers of playing into the pressure to respond to patient's implicit or explicit demands in order to stave off risk of self-destruction:

> If . . . not managed correctly a fixed pattern will evolve in which suicidal threats (or behavior) are used to coerce from others what they must have for psychic survival. Patients such as these must learn other means of getting what they need from others without reflexively threatening death. They are often loathe to learn other means after they have become accustomed to suicidal blackmail and have repeatedly experienced the immediate succor it is likely to produce [p. 203].

By legitimizing or reinforcing self-destructive threats, the therapist risks colluding in re-creating in the group dysfunctional aspects of family dynamics, in which members might fear being overwhelmed by their own inclination to passively force their will on others or perhaps to be victimized by such coercion.[1]

Throughout group, Vivian held firm. She did not negotiate a turn at any point during the session, and she succeeded in commanding considerable control with her silence, as it was difficult to fully concentrate on the work of other members. Although her peers could use their turns to discuss their feelings about Vivian, I could not confront Vivian without taking time from other members who had volunteered to speak.

---

[1]The approach to Vivian I have described here might be considered controversial and risky in the context of standard clinical group practice. My intervention was guided by a calculated willingness to assume "short-term risk" (Maltsberger, 1994) in order to attempt to reduce the long-term threat of more serious self-destructive behavior.

154

When group ended, Vivian likely felt angry and abandoned, as, from her perspective, she was deprived of the time and attention merited by her distress.

When Vivian returned the next day, we learned that she had gone home and cut her arms with a razor. This self-destructive act might have represented an attempt to deal with the emotions and impulses generated by her initial upset as well as a response to possible feelings of abandonment. In terms of its impact on group members, Vivian's self-injury might have functioned either as an expression of aggression or of conflict around aggressive impulses, both of which have been recognized in the literature as motivators for self-destructive behavior (Pao, 1969; M. Friedman et al., 1972; Hull, Lane, and Okie, 1989; Himber, 1994). From this psychodynamic perspective, Vivian's behavior could also be interpreted as an act of retribution. Specifically, by hurting herself, she might have been inflicting upon the group the anger that she had previously refused to verbalize. Perhaps Vivian resisted taking time for herself because she needed to keep in check a greedy and possibly angry inclination to consume all of the group resources (e.g., to talk for the whole session). In this way, self-abnegation may replace negotiation as a means of dealing with limited supplies. The nurturing aspects of self-sacrifice were rendered aggressive by virtue of the absence of active efforts to take care of her own needs. Both the nurturing and the aggressive inclinations became toxic by virtue of their failure to be differentiated from each other. Vivian claimed to be giving something (time) to other group members, but she was actually engaging in an act of aggression as members were put in the position of feeling responsible for her self-inflicted injury by accepting what she offered. Vivian achieved considerable power by avoiding direct verbal expression of her needs in group, as members felt more pressure to respond to her nonverbal distress signals. But this "victory of sorts" came at considerable cost for Vivian, who deprived herself of an opportunity for much needed support and insight, either of which might have helped her to deal more effectively with her distress. She also lost an opportunity to experience others as responding to her without being coerced.

When adolescents offer help or support to others, there is also an opportunity to smuggle aggression into this caregiving role. For example, an adolescent in a psychotherapy group complimented a trainee cotherapist on her new dress and noted that previously the trainee had almost always worn pants or long skirts: "Finally we can see some legs." Although the comment may have appeared to be supportive, the overly enthusiastic tone left the trainee feeling self-conscious about her new look and embarrassed with regard to her more usual dress style. The patient had hit an area of vulnerability, making it difficult for the beginning therapist to explore possible aggressive motives behind the "compliment." Members may collude with one another in undermining therapeutic attempts to confront such covert aggression within the group. For example, when Patient A discloses self-destructive inclinations, Patient B may respond by expressing her sense that she understands A's feelings. B's comment, although framed empathically, shades into provocation for A to act on her impulses. Alternatively, an ostensibly helpful attempt on B's part to confront A about a sensitive area of difficulty may be delivered or pursued with a hint of sadistic relish that could exacerbate A's feeling of vulnerability in the group.

In either of these cases, Patient A may accept the feedback, leaving it to the therapist to confront Patient B. If the therapist does address the hidden aggression, A then may step in to defend B, explaining that B is "just trying to help," and she may proceed to accuse the therapist of unfairly scapegoating B. Now A appears to be taking care of B, when really she is actually undermining an opportunity for B to learn something about herself. The therapist cannot win, because if she decides not to confront B, then A may feel victimized by her passivity and failure to offer protection. A and B might be setting up the therapist to look aggressive so that they can avoid responsibility for their own aggression and their anger toward each other. They may be using shared criticism of the therapist as a basis to bond with each other. Such joint defiance may facilitate the formation of peer relationships at a point when conflict between A and B might jeopardize their developing connection with each other.

This tendency within groups for adolescent or young adult members to join forces against the therapist and undermine therapeutic interventions may also represent a re-creation of the struggle to deal with anger and disappointment toward parents. In the context of the family, a daughter's self-destructive symptoms and lapses in independent functioning can stand as evidence of parental failures. Continued reliance on caregivers for money or for other forms of rescue may express a vengeful wish to drain parents' resources. In an interactive process, parents may willingly sacrifice themselves for adolescent and young adult children as a means of atoning for past failures. In this way, the family system perpetuates a cycle of continued dependence, in which anger is expressed in self-destructive crises, and parents then step in to rescue. In the process, underlying feelings of sadness and anger may be avoided. This circle of vengeance and reparation perpetuates ongoing mutual dependence between parents and adult children, in which a daughter's continued failure to maintain independent functioning provides a sense of purpose for a parent. A daughter can feel powerful despite her dysfunction, because the parent relies on her continued dependence.

The clinical task facing the therapist when these dynamics are played out in group, as in the aforementioned example, is to help the patient explore and direct the anger appropriately. This type of intervention can create the opportunity to face anger and disappointment with the therapist as caregiver while building the capacity to tolerate conflict in supportive peer relationships. Such a clinical process does not happen all at once, and adolescents in particular may need some time to deflect conflict in their peer relationship so as to build a stronger bond before they can directly negotiate anger toward each other. For this reason, episodes like the one described do not necessarily mean that dysfunctional family dynamics have derailed treatment. However, the therapist must also be aware that continued retreat to this type of polarization within the group could represent a form of stagnation, in which dependence is being perpetuated at the expense of developing truly supportive connections with caregivers and peers.

Self-Destructive Behavior as an Expression of Power

Adolescents often feel that autonomy demands self-sufficiency, as opposed to a capacity to seek caregiving in the service of supporting independent functioning. From this perspective, self-destructive behavior may develop as a compromise, serving as a cry for nurturance, "Help me to be safe," and a defiance of protective efforts, "You can't stop me from hurting myself if I want to." Any intervention, then, will inevitably be experienced both as suffocating and inadequate. By rebelling in a self-defeating manner, the adolescent asserts her autonomy while simultaneously dooming progress toward separation, thereby staving off the need to face the loss of parental care and nurturance.

The stance of pseudo–self-sufficiency, "I don't need anything from anyone," allows the adolescent to fend off dependent longings by maintaining an illusion of personal omnipotence. Adolescents often turn to self-destructive behavior to demonstrate their physical and emotional prowess. It feels powerful to reject caregiving and plunge fearlessly into danger. Self-destructive plans may demonstrate strategizing and calculation—skills that, if turned toward achievement, could provide a competitive edge. The self-discipline of an anorectic lifestyle, for example, demonstrates capacity for tenacious, goal-directed effort, evidenced by the consistent food restriction, calorie counting, and rigorous exercise regimes. An illusion of omnipotence is sustained, in part, by avoiding the risk of failure that comes with attempts at competitive achievement. There is, for one thing, more certainty of "success" when the striving takes the form of self-directed behavior. Opposing efforts can be resisted, as no one can control what one does to one's self. The paradox inherent in this struggle was verbalized most clearly by a woman who had been bulimic throughout her young adult years. "When I am going to binge, I am unstoppable. I know the foods I will use to purge, and I become absolutely determined to get them and eat them. I know exactly what I want, and I am determined to get it. With everything else, it's like, well O.K. I wish I knew what I wanted more, and I wish I were more disciplined to achieve goals."

These self-destructive acts can undermine opportunity for real independence. For example, adolescents who have acted on suicidal impulses often become ineligible for structured housing that would allow for a stable, semi-independent lifestyle. These young women are in effect depriving themselves of the best alternative to remaining at home or in a crisis-ridden independent living situation. It is also possible to use self-destructive behavior to mask emotional growth and new potential. For example, when the emerging development of mature sexuality gains expression in the form of promiscuity or unprotected sexual activity, the interpersonal gain and its implications for separation tend to be overshadowed by issues of risk. Therapists and parents then become more afraid to abdicate responsibility to the adolescent, thereby perpetuating childhood dependence.

The Therapist's Emotional Response to Self-Destructive Behavior

When the patient presents as helpless in the face of repeated crises, the therapist must struggle with how much control to try to exert while the adolescent grapples with how much help to accept. To the extent that the therapist takes on the role of the rescuer, the adolescent may become more entrenched in a position of angry, help-rejecting dependence. Or, conversely, the adolescent may submit to the therapist, abdicating control. Although the therapist may feel stressed and burdened by this responsibility, there is also an opportunity here to feel powerful and needed. A pattern of selfless caregiving may be repeated in the treatment relationship, wherein the therapist offers an adolescent help beyond his or her typical parameters. By extending himself or herself in this way, the therapist may be unconsciously identified with the adolescent in her inclination to sacrifice her own needs to care for another, and the adolescent, in turn, might be drawn toward repetition of her experience with her mother's self-sacrifice.

The paradigm of the all-giving helper and the needy other is thereby re-created in the treatment relationship. Polarization in these roles can disguise more complex underlying motives. To what extent does the adolescent's dependence fulfill the therapist's need to be needed? For the adolescent, do the crises and the associated demands for emergency intervention represent an attempt to control and dominate the therapist? For example, when the therapist is awakened by emergency calls and responds only to the adolescent's explicit requests for help, he or she may be colluding with a denial of the adolescent's capacity for aggressive intrusion. In this paradigm, which may be derived from the mother–daughter relationship, recognition of the expression of power and aggression is excluded from a nurturing bond.

By focusing on the adolescent's neediness, the therapist may avoid confronting anger at and disappointment in the adolescent for her intrusive or coercive demands. Threats of self-destructive behavior, for example, may be used to try to dictate the behavior and availability of the therapist (e.g., "I need to call you in the evening to keep from cutting myself"). An attempt on the part of the therapist to remain unruffled may communicate, in effect, that he or she is so powerful as to be untouched by the adolescent's most desperate attempts to make an emotional impact. By embracing the adolescent's apparent dependence in this way, the therapist diminishes the adolescent's power. If the therapist denies the emotional impact of such provocative demands, the adolescent is disarmed. This could result in an escalation of aggression in the form of more dangerous behavior or a turn toward increased dependence in which autonomy is (perhaps aggressively) forsaken in favor of reliance on the therapist, who may become increasingly idealized. If the therapist fails to recognize the adolescent's aggression, issues of power, competition, and coercion in the treatment relationship cannot be confronted in face-to-face conflict.

Neither the therapist nor the patient, then, has to deal with the therapist's anger at the patient or with the patient's anger or disappointment in the therapist. Such confrontations could over time foster increased mutuality and intimacy, as the two together grapple with the limits of the therapist's power to protect, the patient's conflicts about asking for help, her fears of being turned down, the therapist's reactions to the different ways that the patient seeks help, and the meaning to each of the adolescent's increasing capacity for autonomy. The competitive, angry, empathic, aggressive, fearful, playful, or vulnerable moments that surface in the course of such interaction could allow for a more multidimensional experience of a caregiving relationship. The following discussion considers ways that such new interpersonal experience can provide a forum for the adolescent to venture beyond the confines of historically familiar roles with a caregiver and to discover and express more of who she is in her own right.

Implications for the Therapeutic Relationship

When an adolescent perceives her mother as selfless, she may feel more guilty about her anger and frustration with their relationship, her need to break away, and her own "selfishness" or other shortcomings as a developing caregiver. The therapist, in turn, may be pressured by the adolescent's expectations for similarly selfless caregiving in treatment as well as his or her own aspirations to deliver some form of healing nurturance. I would argue, however, that it is in this effort to assert his or her limitations that the therapist can often best support the adolescent's autonomy and offer an opportunity for a more balanced experience with caregiving. For example, by acknowledging that he or she cannot stop the adolescent from hurting herself, the therapist is recognizing the adolescent's responsibility for her own life. Furthermore, by admitting that limits exist with regard to his or her ability to nurture, the therapist challenges the illusion of selfless caregiving. In this process, the therapist is acknowledging that his or her needs may compete or conflict with those of the adolescent.

In work with adults, the therapist's needs are introduced automatically into treatment through issues around payment, but these financial demands may be more distant or abstract for adolescents or young adults whose therapy is funded by parents. However, even beyond such treatment parameters, the adolescent and the therapist must reckon with the reality that there are bounds to what the therapist can give emotionally and that there is also therapeutic value to limiting the therapist's availability and involvement. Perhaps most challenging to our identity as therapists is the recognition that there is also a limit to what we are willing to give, even if the giving would be good for the adolescent, instead of bad for her. Yes, by offering the adolescent an experience of caregiving balanced by self-interest, the therapist might provide a positive role model. But that is not the point. If the therapist rationalizes the personal limits he or she sets as being entirely for the patient's benefit, then neither the therapist nor the patient can come to grips with the place of self-interest and separateness in the caregiving relationship.

In the process of setting these limits, the therapist is also implicitly recognizing the adolescent's capacity for independent functioning. It is critical in work with adolescents to attend to strivings for autonomy as well as longings for dependence, so that both sides of the conflict around separation are brought into the therapy. In this way, the therapeutic relationship can help to promote the integration of these seemingly irreconcilable emotional needs. From this perspective, the therapist would need to recognize the progressive, autonomous strivings embodied in the self-destructive behavior without supporting or sanctioning the action itself. In addition, the therapist must recognize the aggression in his or her own angry response to the adolescent's demands and provocations or, alternatively, the aggression in denying the impact of the adolescent's provocations.

To illustrate some of the complexity and ambiguity inherent in this therapeutic stance, I present a clinical example of a power struggle with a 21-year-old woman that developed during the termination phase of a partial hospitalization treatment for which I served as the individual therapist. The therapeutic conflict centered on risk associated with this young woman's emerging sexuality. The patient, whom I call Chris here, had been referred to the program because of her history of self-destructive behavior, which included severe anorexia, alcohol abuse, overdosing on prescribed medications, cutting her wrists, and several near-lethal suicide attempts that required hospitalization. She had also been injured repeatedly in the course of her sports involvement and would continue to play before she had healed. In this way, she had caused a serious chronic neck injury. About a year into treatment, I learned from other staff that Chris had initiated a sexual relationship with a man diagnosed with bipolar disorder and mild mental retardation, whom I call Steve, whom she had met on an inpatient psychiatric unit when she was a teenager. She had contracted herpes early on in their sexual encounters, as Steve had failed to inform her of his condition and take adequate precautions. Before this, she had had only one sexual experience, which took the form of one-time, unprotected intercourse with a young man who was a stranger to her. Throughout the early phases of treatment, I had repeatedly confronted Chris about her secretiveness regarding her potentially dangerous behaviors. For example, on hot summer days she would sometimes appear with long sleeves to hide bandages on her arms that covered self-inflicted cuts. I would learn of vomiting and laxative abuse only if I noticed and inquired about swelling in her face. Chris was obviously ambivalent about keeping her self-destructive behavior hidden, because the long sleeves and the edema functioned to attract my attention. I would venture interpretations about her secrecy, as well as the ensuing pattern of interaction, in which her passivity in the face of potential danger would make me want to "drag" information out of her and try to frighten her into protective action. Specifically, I wondered with Chris whether my experience of myself as heavy-handed and intrusive in these interactions might have represented a repetition of prior experience with caregivers. I also wondered about her role in creating this type of distrustful interaction, and, specifically, I questioned what drew her toward this position, in which she would feel pursued and pressured to disclose facets of her personal life. I had come to regard her silence and avoidance as a danger sign, and I felt concerned about her attempt to hide from me her new sexual relationship. At the same time, I found it hard to differentiate Chris's inclination to hide self-destructive behavior from a wish for privacy, and I wanted to be respectful of her need to maintain her own separate life.

I told Chris that I had learned of her new relationship from other staff, and I wondered with her about her decision not to tell me herself. She responded with continued evasiveness and silence, my concern and irritation intensified, and I felt more inclined to challenge her avoidance and to probe for information about possible hidden danger. I acknowledged her recent progress with self-care, but I also confronted her with my anger and fear that she might again be failing to protect herself from possible exposure to sexually transmitted disease. She said nothing to reassure me or to show that she even emotionally registered the risk. Chris seemed to be selectively attuned to my frustration, and she experienced my concern and efforts to protect her solely as criticism. I did not back down, but I acknowledged that I appreciated her autonomy with regard to her behavior as well as self-disclosure. Her involvement with Steve continued, and she mentioned her plans to move into his apartment when she entered a program to train and work part-time as a computer programmer. This would involve a move away from the neighborhood where her parents and extended family all resided in close proximity. Although I questioned the timing of the move relative to her readiness to leave structured housing, I did not oppose her. I continued to feel uneasy about her welfare, but I also suspected that, in choosing to disclose her sexual involvement to staff, Chris expected that I would learn of it. She also knew, based on past experience in treatment, that I would be attuned to health issues and would likely confront her. I asked Chris whether the focus on issues of risk around her sexual behavior might be a distraction from emotional dangers in the relationship. In response, she opened up a bit and began to talk about Steve's difficulty with commitment. She explained that sometimes he would be enthusiastic about living together, whereas other times he would tell her he wanted to leave her.

Several weeks later, Chris told me that she had felt hurt by my disapproval of her involvement with Steve, which, she said, made it difficult for her to talk freely with me. I was like her high-powered professional parents, she said, in that I never felt satisfied with her. I told her that I did not disapprove of the relationship and that, in fact, I knew little about Steve. I confronted her, in turn, about the fact that she had told me many disturbing and worrisome things about Steve while sharing little of what she liked about him. Then, she had turned around and criticized me for not accepting him. She laughed. This was a moment of connection in which we could relate genuinely, letting go of our familiar roles. With this laugh, Chris was acknowledging that she had a role in our cat-and-mouse pattern of interaction.

Chris began to talk of the pain she felt in her relationship with Steve. With his limited capacity to tolerate sustained intimacy, Steve would open himself emotionally to Chris, and, as they began to experience a deepened sense of closeness, he would withdraw and sometimes even adopt a rejecting stance. I wondered if, by committing herself to Steve, she might be repeating patterns from her family in which she dedicated her emotional energy to people who had serious problems. She said that that might be the case but that she did not want more intimacy because it was too overwhelming. She explained that she did not really think that Steve would leave her, that she loved being with him, and that he was pursuing psychiatric treatment and taking medication. At the time, she was preparing to leave the partial hospital program and her residential situation. She wanted to live with him, perhaps marry him.

As far as I could tell, Chris was beginning to let go of her overtly self-destructive behaviors. But her continued reticence and secretiveness had helped to perpetuate a polarization in our relationship, in which I was the vigilant, suspicious one, on guard for self-imposed danger, and she placidly embraced worrisome developments in her life. I cannot be sure whether Chris felt abandoned when I confronted the limits of my control over her involvement with Steve. Up to that point, each step she made toward autonomy seemed to pose a risk for compensatory self-destructive regression. As Chris had progressed toward termination, it became more difficult to know whether there were self-destructive elements to her choices or whether they were merely different from the choices that I might have wished for her. It is possible that Chris wanted me to feel dubious, as it would likely have been more difficult for her to leave me if I could more fully embrace her choices. Maybe she needed to see that I could stay involved with her even if she challenged and rejected me. It is also possible that Chris had really wanted me to intercede in her plans because she could not stop herself from including a self-destructive component in her ventures toward independence.

The ambiguity surrounding Chris's choices likely reflected some intermingling of regressive and progressive motives as well as self-defeating and self-empowering inclinations. That I could not stop her from acting self-destructively and that I could not even know, with any certainty, whether her choices were self-destructive drove home the reality of Chris's autonomy and her separateness in our relationship. In the course of my confrontations and our conflict, I was not able to feel entirely confident about her safety. I shared with Chris my appreciation for the growth in her personal life, but I also acknowledged my concern that, in supporting her involvement with Steve, I might be letting her down by failing to recognize hidden dangers. By disclosing both sides of my experience of Chris at this juncture in her treatment and in her life, I found myself more able to continue feeling close and invested as I began to emotionally let go.

As in my work with Chris, the process by which the therapist is able to abdicate responsibility for the adolescent's decision making is a function of the complex and intangible dynamics of therapeutic interaction. The therapist, like the parent, cannot achieve a perfect balance of protective control and trusting respect for autonomy. It is therefore necessary for the therapist to recognize the lack of purity of his or her own motives—specifically, to remain aware that competitive, self-protective, and aggressive feelings, as well as personal identification with the adolescent, may mingle with inclinations to nurture the adolescent's individual identity and values. If the existence of aggression in a caregiving relationship can be recognized and acknowledged, the press for the adolescent to express her anger in the form of self-destructive behavior is reduced.

The integration of nurturance and aggression on the part of the therapist provides a different and more balanced model of caregiving, perhaps allowing the adolescent to differentiate this experience from her struggle to separate from her mother. The therapist must also grapple with the meaning of the separation for himself or herself, as well as the implications of the adolescent's power for self-determination in the treatment relationship. For example, to the extent that the therapist feels a sense of superior wisdom and judgment or a sense of personal empowerment to protect in the relationship with the adolescent, such experience may carry over into his or her own life, functioning to reduce feelings of vulnerability. Only by accepting the dangers presented by self-destructive behavior and the therapist's own limitations in protecting the adolescent is there opportunity for the young woman to accept and embrace both the destructive and constructive potential of her own aggressive and autonomous strivings. The adolescent can then turn from self-imposed risk to face and engage with risks in the world outside of the family orbit.

REFERENCES

Almqvist, F. (1986), Sex differences in adolescent psychopathology. *Acta Psychiat. Scand.*, 73:295–306.

Benjamin, J. (1991), Father and daughter: Identification with difference—A contribution to gender heterodoxy. *Psychoanal. Dial.*, 1:277–300.

Bernstein, G. A., Garfinkel, B. D. & Hoberman, H. M. (1989), Self-reported anxiety in adolescents. *Amer. J. Psychiat.*, 146:384–386.

Chodorow, N. (1978), *The Reproduction of Mothering.* Berkeley: University of California Press.

——— (1989), *Feminism and Psychoanalytic Theory*. New Haven, CT: Yale University Press.

Dimen, M. (1991), Deconstructing difference: Gender, splitting, and transitional space. *Psychoanal. Dial.*, 1:335–352.

Friedman, G. (1980), The mother–daughter bond. *Contemp. Psychoanal.*, 16:90–97.

Friedman, M., Glasser, M., Laufer E., Laufer M. & Wohl, M. (1972), Attempted suicide and self-mutilation in adolescence: Some observations from a psychoanalytic research project. *Internat. J. Psychoanal.*, 53:179–183.

Goldner, V. (1991), Toward a critical relational theory of gender. *Psychoanal. Dial.*, 1:249–272.

Hendin, H. (1981), Psychotherapy and suicide. *Amer. J. Psychother.*, 35:469–480.

Himber, J. (1994), Blood rituals: Self-cutting in female psychiatric inpatients. *Psychother.*, 31:620–631.

Horner, A. (1991), From idealization to ideal—From attachment to identification: The female analyst and the female patient. *J. Amer. Acad. Psychoanal.*, 18:223–232.

Hull, J. W., Lane, R. C. & Okie, J. (1989), Sexual acting out and the desire for revenge. *Psychoanal. Rev.*, 76:313–328.

Jordan, J. V., Kaplan, A. G., Miller, J. B., Stiver, I. P. & Surrey, J. L. (1991), *Women's Growth in Connection*. New York: Guilford.

Kaftal, E. (1991), On intimacy between men. *Psychoanal. Dial.*, 1:305–328.

Kashani, J. H., Beck, N. C., Hoeper, E. W., Fallahi, C., Corcoran, C. M., McAllister, J. A., Rosenberg, T. K. & Reid, J. C. (1987), Psychiatric disorders in a sample of adolescents. *Amer. J. Psychiat.*, 144:584–589.

Leadbeater, B. J., Blatt, S. J. & Quinlan, D. M. (1995), Gender-linked vulnerabilities to depressive symptoms, stress, and problem behaviors in adolescents. *J. Res. Adoles.*, 5:1–29.

Maltsberger, J. T. (1994), Calculated risks in the treatment of intractably suicidal patients. *Psychiat.*, 57:199–212.

Miller, J. B. (1991), The construction of anger in women and men. In: *Women's Growth in Connection*, ed. J. V. Jordan, A. G. Kaplan, J. B. Miller, I. P. Stiver & J. L. Surrey. New York: Guilford, pp. 181–196.

Pao, P. (1969), The syndrome of delicate self-cutting. *Brit. J. Medical Psychol.*, 42:195–206.

Schonert-Reichl, K. A. & Offer, D. (1992), Gender differences in adolescent symptoms. In: *Advances in Clinical Child Psychology*, ed. B. B. Lahey & A. E. Kazdin. New York: Plenum Press, pp. 27–60.

Spezzano, C. (1993), *Affect in Psychoanalysis*. Hillsdale, NJ: The Analytic Press.

PART IV

SCHOOL-BASED AND PREVENTIVE PROGRAMS

For most adolescents in our culture, school is their natural habitat. It is there that their cognitive skills are sharpened, their social relationships forged, and their affective (and sexual) experiences largely focused. This being the case, it would seem that the school is a logical and appropriate site for mental health interventions, both preventive and therapeutic. The chapters in this section address both the potentialities and the problems attendant upon such efforts. Domeena Renshaw, a noted authority on sex education for teenagers, updates us on the vital issue of adolescents and AIDS and proposes approaches to prevention based both on the school and on other community resources. Gary Mauk and Jim Sharpnack consider the equally troubling problem of adolescent suicide. They describe a successful program geared to the needs of peer and classmate survivors in such situations. Glen Pearson and his colleagues present a comprehensive system of school-based mental health services in a large urban community, setting forth both its successes and the administrative difficulties they have encountered in developing and implementing it. Finally, Richard Gottlieb discusses the special problems of providing psychotherapy to boarding school students and tells how recent developments in the broader field of health policy have transformed, and largely impeded, the possibility of doing so at this time.

A special section on school-based services is planned for our next volume.

9 ADOLESCENT SEX AND AIDS

DOMEENA C. RENSHAW

In my 1987 article, "AIDS and Sexuality," my final paragraph was: "Has AIDS changed dating and mating behavior? The answer is both yes and no. This is only the opening chapter of AIDS knowledge. We need at least another decade to see the impact of the most vigorous research and sex education campaign in history" (p. 37).

By 1997, the explosion of AIDS information in print and electronically from that campaign has become overwhelming in volume but far less impressive in research design, quality, and clarity. A vital fact is that, in most states, only AIDS and not HIV-positive cases are reportable to public health authorities. Therefore, we have only estimates of the HIV-positive cases. Millions of allotted research dollars were spent to provide widespread bilingual education on AIDS preventive measures (defined as condom use, abstinence, or delayed first intercourse). AIDS risk behaviors were measured mostly by questionnaire or an interview before and after an administered AIDS education program. Did adolescents learn about the risks of unprotected sex, alcohol, or drug abuse? Outcomes were unclear, and the reading level of the teens was not mentioned. Could they understand the questionnaires? Literally hundreds of very similar teen surveys have been done. Were the dollars well spent? In many studies, the answer is no. It would have been much more medically useful had serological HIV blood tests been done instead of or in addition to the surveys.

The state of California funded a large, 1992–1994 program, "Postponing Sexual Involvement," to reduce adolescent pregnancy. Education, given to 187,000 teens in 31 counties, consisted of five sessions dealing with why teens have sex, the risks of pregnancy and sexually transmitted diseases, and why teens should wait until marriage for sex (abstinence only). In a careful review (Alan Guttmacher Institute, 1994), this education program showed no impact at all on adolescent sex behavior. A family planning council funded the review by Douglas Kirby and mentioned that the teens in this program had not been given contraceptive information. As a result, the program closed. Internal and public politics subsequently protested, because the Guttmacher Institute allegedly had received donations from the same family planning council that requested Kirby's study. Petty as all this may sound, politics continues to play a significant role in many funded educational efforts that aim to prevent both AIDS and teen pregnancy.

Adolescence is a transitional phase. Containing it is as difficult as capturing a cloud pattern. Studies struggle with complex physical, emotional, and social factors. Puberty is a time of the highest level of circulating sex hormones and arousal, but it is also a time of magical thinking, feeling both anxious and invulnerable, behaving impulsively, having low sexual controls and little awareness of consequences, and having few social skills and little understanding of the body changes that are occurring. Experiments with driving, sex, smoking, sports, drugs, and alcohol all are going on. Learning and reading disorders as well as some disabilities (deafness, blindness) may make it more difficult to understand the content when sex and AIDS education programs are given. Meantime, the whole population is regularly and repeatedly imploded with provocative sexual images via television, videos, magazines, billboards, and the Internet. Marketing anything is enhanced by sex symbols. Sudden normal reflex erections are common in male teens. This sometimes can be embarrassing (Mayle, 1975). Reflex arousal can also occur normally in girls (clitoral throbbing and lubrication). Only rarely will an adolescent ask a grown-up about these reactions. If he or she tells a peer, there may be unexpected consequences such as spreading hurtful rumors or being openly ridiculed. Many teens feel very alone and confused about their sex reactions. Accurate sex education can provide great relief simply by informing them that they are normal (Mayle and Robins, 1981). A library or the Internet may be explored. Copycat behavior is another way to learn, whether about break-dancing or about sex, but the risks are different.

Experimentation is a normal way to learn. Teens try out driving, cigarettes, alcohol, drugs, and meeting new peers, often simultaneously. They explore strange haircuts, dress, music, dance, and other activities. They protest restrictions by parents and teachers. Lying, rebellion, and ridicule become "cool" and an avenue to form bonds with peers doing the same. This can cause multiple family crises, particularly if a pregnancy, a car crash, or venereal disease results from trial-and-error learning. Adolescent driving lessons are easily accepted by nearly all parents and schools, yet lessons on sex and sexually transmitted diseases may evoke parental withholding of the teen's attendance. Yet, no sex education is sex education. No sex education says that this family or school finds discussing sex too difficult.

An important professional or medical question is how severe is the U.S. teen AIDS problem. The answer depends on where the figures were obtained. Loosely, it is estimated that 1:80 teenage boys and 1:500 girls were HIV positive in 1997. These are not AIDS cases but HIV positives. They are also estimates and may be inaccurate. The *Morbidity and Mortality Weekly Report* (Centers for Disease Control and Prevention, 1996a) summarizes U.S. 1994 AIDS figures: total, 78,279; under 1 year, 318; 1 to 4 years, 418; 5 to 9 years, 148; 10 to 14 years, 146; 15 to 19 years, 324; and 30 to 39 years, 35,466 (the largest cluster).

In the *HIV/AIDS Surveillance Report* through December 1996 (Centers for Disease Control and Prevention, 1996b), cumulative U.S. AIDS cases were as follows: under 5 years, 6,032; 5 to 12 years, 1,597; and 13 to 19 years, 2,754. Although not trivializing the problem, in an adolescent population of more than 24 million, these figures do not seem of epidemic or pandemic proportions. However, because HIV-positive status may be detected as many as 10 years before AIDS-positive status, it is said that "new" cases in 20- to 29-year-olds were possibly contracted during adolescence. Unreported HIV-positive cases are unknown because they are not reportable in most states. A recent concern is that, in the 3 years since 1992, girl adolescent AIDS figures doubled and may continue to rise despite the use of anti-AIDS combination medication and hopes of a vaccine. An oft-repeated figure is a 330% increase in the number of AIDS cases in 13- to 19-year-olds between 1988 and 1994—from 325 to 1,070 cases. The 1996 figure already mentioned was 2,754 in 24 million. There are several sets of tables, not easy to sort out by clinicians.

For each child and family, one member's infection with AIDS is one too many and a major tragedy. Adolescent pregnancy is a shock for an individual and a family, but is it comparable to an impending AIDS death? There is much posturing and politics by conservative groups regarding both teen pregnancy and AIDS. No one disagrees that both conditions are social and personal problems. Groups who oppose sex education argue that prevention-of-pregnancy programs are perceived as permission for teens to have premarital sex, whereas abstinence-only programs could have (perhaps) prevented the coital consequences of both pregnancy and AIDS. However, the reality is that biosociocultural changes in the late 1990s show earlier puberty, better health, more spending money, improved overall education, and marriage at a later age than in the 1940s. More families now have two working parents or one parent and less adult/parental supervision. Adolescents explore their sexuality earlier, in cars, at home alone, or wherever else they like. Do teens do the opposite of what adults suggest? Often, yes. Should authorities then give up on AIDS prevention and sex/pregnancy/contraception education? Definitely not. Many teaching techniques have been tried—theater, rehearsal role-playing, lectures, videos, comics, pamphlets—but the outcomes of most have not been reported. One controlled study of theater in AIDS education reports little impact on before-and-after knowledge and attitudes (Elliot et al., 1996). Before-and-after questionnaires test immediate memory, not integration and behavioral changes.

Would peer AIDS educators, trained and paid, be more acceptable, as teens are the principal sex educators of teens? Yes. The WEDGE program in San Francisco has people with AIDS (PWAs) talk to adolescents and allow them to ask questions. Are PWAs dismissed as "goody two-shoes" and part of the "grown-up" sector? Usually not. As AIDS- or HIV-positive teen educators, are they effective? Usually. Could this backfire, as with Magic Johnson, who is active, athletic, employed, traveling, wealthy, a star in the news? Perhaps, because some may think, "AIDS is not so bad after all." Therefore, teen educators nearly always state that very fact, "You may not believe me because I look okay now, but I have AIDS, and I want to help others not to get infected."

Hemophilic adolescent males are said to comprise 44% of reported AIDS cases in U.S. male teenage groups. These males passively contracted AIDS from clotting factors in donated blood for the treatment of their congenital bleeding illness before organizations started testing these products for AIDS. Hemophilic teens are today usually well informed regarding AIDS. In the sexually active segment of these AIDS-positive hemophilics, however, only 31% told their partner of their infection, stating fear of rejection by the partner (Forsberg et al., 1996). Counselors were making the extra effort to educate them by rehearsing how to inform the partner and how to use condoms to lessen the risk to the partner. An interesting fact was noted. Although 75% of U.S. sex curricula mentioned use of condoms, only 9% included information of how to apply and remove condoms. Adolescents need to learn and be confident in how to use condoms if and when they decide to be sexually active.

Males and Chew (1996) researched fathers who had impregnated adolescent girls and found that 41% of one cluster of 518,000 U.S. adolescent mothers omitted the name of the child's father. In its study of 70,000 teen births, the California Center for Health Statistics (CCHS) reported that most of the fathers were not age-matched peers but were men 5 to 10 years older. This raises speculation as to whether the infants in both studies may have been conceived from rape, incest or sex abuse. The teen mothers may have been fearful of identifying the father. Although the CCHS survey did not study HIV-positive or AIDS cases, it is mentioned to heighten awareness that a pregnancy is not always consensual, particularly in minors, and so HIV testing is essential to caring for both mother and infant.

What comes through clearly in the hundreds of funded high school studies is that much ignorance remains about AIDS, even in affluent neighborhoods. Prevalent myths are that urinating after intercourse lessens risk, donating blood can lead to AIDS, condoms can be reused, and so forth. The length of the questionnaires (79 or 150 questions) seems to challenge the attention span of teens. Most conclude that more study is needed because outcomes are confusing or so varied.

For the clinician, it is practical to be aware of this. Further, adolescents' responses may change as they attempt to sort out their thinking, gather more information, and experience normal mood fluctuations.

An outline of AIDS risk factors for teens includes sexual intercourse with an HIV-positive or AIDS partner, with a homeless person or other stranger, with a prostitute, combined with alcohol/marijuana use, while having a sexually transmitted disease, with multiple sexual partners, unprotected (voluntary/coercive; heterosexual or homosexual), while incarcerated, and during sexual exploitation (rape, incest, child abuse). Nonsexual causes of AIDS infection are AIDS-positive mother, hemophilia treatment, intravenous drug use, and needle sticks in a health care setting.

Sources for AIDS education and treatment are available and are within the reach of parents, teachers, concerned adults, and the teens themselves. It is truly unnecessary for the reckless to get more reckless about AIDS in the 1990s (Renshaw, 1987). Confidential phone calls can be made on a toll-free (800) line; callers need not give their names but can listen and obtain information, direction, and guidance. Some resources have a hotline with volunteers who answer questions. Special efforts have been made to run programs not only at schools but also through Street Outreach AIDS programs for the many teen dropouts, in public housing and in the inner city for minorities, and even in shopping malls for drug abusers, migrants, runaways, and homeless teens. Juvenile offenders have also received AIDS sex education efforts in jails and prisons. AIDS outreach centers and clinics are in the white pages of the telephone book under *AIDS* (see Appendix).

Important wholesome sex education principles for every child and teen must be repeatedly provided by parent, teacher, counselor, minister, or physician. For emphasis, these are outlined:

1. Every human (boy or girl) has normal sexual feelings that come and go, day or night—even during sleep. There may be sexual dreams, sleep erections, sleep orgasms for both sexes, and wet dreams (ejaculate in sleep). These are natural and normal.

2. It is healthy, natural, and normal to enjoy closeness and wanting to be held. Touching feels good, and prolonged touching can lead to sexual arousal. This can be pleasurable, exciting, sometimes "scary" because powerful. Stop then, if you do not want intercourse. Say firmly, "No, stop. This is enough." The excitement will subside in a few minutes. Both partners have to live with consequences if they have impulsive intercourse. Brief moments of delight need not go all the way. It is a decision to do so or a decision to stop.

3. Having sex is not the same as making love. Many people get mixed up about this important difference. There can be lots of love without sex. There is also a lot of sex with no love at all. Hurt and violence can get mixed in with sex, and disease or death may follow. This is scary. Most persons want sex to be good, romantic, and all pleasure. A bad outcome is not just grown-up talk to upset kids. Both girl and boy teens get confused when sex goes bad. Many adolescents say they feel pressure from their peers to have sex before they are ready.

4. A grown-up to talk to may help. Mother, father, a teacher, a pastor, or a physician may be surprised to hear the questions, but they will listen and will help to find answers.

5. Some books combine humor and accurate sex education to help teens to learn and to talk about this important everyday topic (Mayle, 1975; Mayle and Robins, 1981).

176

Improved treatment for AIDS has not as yet proved curative, so potential lethality remains high even with protease inhibiting drugs. The United Nations and the World Health Organization are alarmed that 3 million people became infected with HIV worldwide in 1996, that Africa is the region hardest hit, and that Russia, China, and Brazil are also now affected.

In summary, the current U.S. connection among sex, AIDS, and teenagers has been reviewed. Contradictory reports cause confusion. Useful findings need extraction from the mountain of funded surveys and opinion polls (rather than serological tests) now in the literature. Clinicians and others charged with protecting teens from impulsive sexual actions must learn as much as is available. The question remains unanswered as to whether there was a U.S. teen HIV-positive crisis in 1997.

Teenagers are a precious resource. They are the future of any society. In the United States, more efforts and resources are directed than anywhere in the world to help adolescents avoid the dangers of sexually transmitted diseases, AIDS, and unwanted pregnancy. The task is complicated due to teens' transition toward independence and self-direction. The goal is to provide useful education that teens can absorb and use to protect the self from negative aspects of sexual activity. Each teen must learn to understand, enjoy, and protect natural sexual expression. Learning to relate closely to another—to build closeness, trust, loyalty, and love—will then become the vital context for making a commitment later with mutuality and maturity.

REFERENCES

Alan Guttmacher Institute (1994), *Sex and America's Teenagers*. New York: Alan Guttmacher Institute.

Centers for Disease Control and Prevention (1996a), AIDS associated with injecting-drug use—United States, 1995. *Morbidity & Mortality Wkly. Rep.*, 45:392–398.

———— (1996b), *HIV/AIDS Surveillance Report*. Atlanta, GA: Centers for Disease Control and Prevention.

Elliot, L., Gruer, L., Farrow, K., Henderson, A. & Cowan, L. (1996), Theatre in AIDS education—A controlled study. *AIDS Care*, 8:321–340.

Forsberg, A. D., King, G., Delaronde, S. R., Geary, M. K. & Hemophilia Behavioral Evaluative Intervention Project Committee. (1996),

Maintaining safer sex behaviors in HIV-infected adolescents with hemophilia. *AIDS Care*, 8:629–640.

Males, M. A. & Chew, K. S. Y. (1996), The age of fathers in California adolescent births. *Amer. J. Public Health,* 86:565–568.

Mayle, P. (1975), *What's Happening to Me?* Melbourne, Australia: Sun Books.

———— & Robins, A. (1981), *Congratulations You're Not Pregnant.* New York: Macmillan.

Renshaw, D. C. (1987), AIDS and sexuality. *Proc. Inst. Med. Chicago*, 40(2):36–37.

Appendix

- Counselors at the 24-hr *CDC National HIV/AIDS Hotline* (1-800-342-AIDS) will answer questions, provide basic information and the name of the nearest place to get a confidential HIV test, and send CDC publications by mail (about 3 weeks).
- The Spanish-speaking *CDC National SIDA Hotline* (1-800-344-7432) is available from 8 a.m. to 2 p.m. EST every day.
- The *CDC National TTY Hotline for the Hearing Impaired* (1-800-243-7889) is available 10 a.m. to 10 p.m. EST Monday through Friday.
- *NAPA (National Association of People with AIDS),* operates a volunteer-staffed, 24-hr confidential hotline (1-800-838-9990).
- The teen-staffed *Teens Teaching AIDS Prevention (Teens TAP) Hotline* (1-800-234-8336) is available 4 p.m. to 8 p.m. CST Monday through Friday.
- Callers with fax machines can obtain hundreds of publications from the *National AIDS Clearinghouse FAX Service* (1-800-458-5231, ext. 7091).
- The *CDC National AIDS Clearinghouse* operates a Web site (http://www.cdcnac.org).
- *AEGIS (AIDS Education and Global Information System)* and *HIV/Net* operate a Web site (http://www.hivnet.org) that features downloadable AIDS-related newsletters and education/prevention information.

10   A LIGHT UNTO THE DARKNESS:

THE PSYCHOEDUCATIONAL IMPERATIVE

OF SCHOOL-BASED SUICIDE POSTVENTION

GARY W. MAUK AND JIM D. SHARPNACK

School is where we equip children for life, and loss is part of life
[Turner, 1996, p. 1].

To be human in the world is to experience loss, and children and adolescents encounter loss quite frequently in their lives from a variety of expected and unexpected causes (Hundley and Bratton, 1994; Schonfeld, Kline, and Members of the Crisis Intervention Committee, 1994; Turner, 1996; Mauk and Sharpnack, 1997). Oates (1993) asserted, "If one adds to the deaths of parents and relatives the increasing number of violent deaths of school-age children, it seems unlikely that any school-age child will reach adulthood without experiencing a loss related to death" (p. 38). For example, a study of middle-school students in North Carolina revealed that more than 40% of the students had been personally involved with death within the past year (Glass, 1991).

Unfortunately, however, as James and Cherry (1988) observed, "we are better prepared to deal with minor accidents than we are to deal with the grief caused by death. Simple first aid gets more attention in our world than death and emotional loss" (p. 12). The suicide of an individual, especially a young person, is an anomalous and tragic event, and young people who experience and who are aggrieved by the death of a peer, friend, or acquaintance by suicide are often in crisis (Valente and Saunders, 1993; Mauk and Rodgers, 1994).

Dunn and Morrish-Vidners (1987–1988) observed that the difficult task of suicide bereavement is complicated further by the social stigma surrounding suicide and the uncertainty, confusion, and awkwardness

179

of other individuals' reactions to the event. They further observed, "Recovery from this type of loss thus threatens to be delayed by numerous emotional and social impediments faced by the survivor" (p. 176). Finally, Cimbolic and Jobes (1990) stated, "While it is clear that survivors can and do cope with this awful legacy, education and training of both survivors and interventionists can only facilitate the grief work survivors must undertake" (p. 83).

Suicide and Schools in the United States

The rate of suicide among young people in the United States has tripled since 1950, and Blau (1996) noted disturbingly that "children aged 10 to 14 are killing themselves three times more often than they did 20 years ago" (p. 188). For 1995, the most recent aggregate data reporting year, the National Center for Health Statistics (Anderson, Kochanek, and Murphy, 1997) reported that, among 5- to 14-year-olds (all races, both sexes), there was a total of 337 suicidal deaths (0.9 per 100,000), and, among 15- to 24-year-olds (all races, both sexes), a total of 4,956 suicidal deaths (13.8 per 100,000). Accordingly, this makes suicide the sixth and third leading causes of death among youth ages 5 to 14 and 15 to 24, respectively, in the United States.

Suicide is not something that happens only in someone else's school or school district. In contemporary America, all schools are at risk for crises such as the suicide of a student (Berman and Jobes, 1991; Poland, 1995; Poland, Pitcher, and Lazarus, 1995; Sandoval and Brock, 1996). Very few schools, especially secondary schools, have escaped the tragedy of adolescent suicide and its devastating impact on the school community (Capuzzi, 1994; Celotta, 1995). Unfortunately, sooner or later educators who work with young people will experience and have to deal with the problem of suicide.

However, the tragedy of the suicide of a child or adolescent has more than one victim (Carter and Brooks, 1990; Renaud, 1995). The death usually leaves behind a myriad of survivors who must live in the psychosocially tumultuous wake of the event (Dunne, 1992). For every adolescent suicide, there is a minimum of three additional people (e.g., peers, family members) who are so affected by this violent death that "the resulting traumatic reactions claim their lives by burdening them with such intense reactions that they suffer cognitively, socially, psychologically, and emotionally" (Steele, 1992, p. 17). The suicide of a peer is a particularly toxic form of death for the surviving friends and acquaintances (Mauk and Weber, 1991).

The Death of a Peer by Suicide

"Suicide is a mode of death that is mostly experienced as a brutal dissolution of life, and a violent disunion of existing relationships" (Cleiren and Diekstra, 1995, p. 7). As such, young people who are friends and classmates of a deceased peer are indirect victims, subject to survivor guilt manifested in physical and psychosomatic illness, depression, or acting out, especially anger (Kliman, 1978; Brent et al., 1992; Brent et al., 1993; Valente and Saunders, 1993). Many adolescents are affected by the death of a peer, but their grief may be ignored because the main priority of the bereavement process is on surviving family members (Raphael, 1983). In fact, peer bereavement during childhood and adolescence is often a matter of "disenfranchised grief" (Doka, 1989, p. 4), and young people who are bereaved over a peer's or friend's death are often "forgotten grievers," who are seldom given appropriate attention as they struggle to cope with their loss (Doka, 1989).

Adolescent suicide is a particularly disturbing mode of death for friends and acquaintances who are left behind in its wake (Mauk and Rodgers, 1994). Suicide is a self-administered, separate, and distinct cause of death that cannot be compared to any other crisis (Tanney, 1995). Further, the stigma and proscription that exist regarding suicide serve to intensify the survivors' feelings of blame, self-doubt, confusion, shame, resentment, and guilt (Dunne, 1992). For the adolescent survivor, who views the self as indestructible, the death of a friend or acquaintance challenges his or her coping resiliency (Mauk and Weber, 1991). In most cases, survivors will have little time for anticipatory grief (Cleiren and Diekstra, 1995).

Trauma-Induced Psychological Disequilibrium and Postvention Services for Student Survivors of Suicide

Students in the schools of the 1990s unfortunately are quite familiar with peers who die by accidents, homicide, and suicide (Blom, Etkind, and Carr, 1991; Deaton and Berkan, 1995). Such familiarity places the issues of suicide and other modes of death into the school environment and into the realm of educators and other adults who themselves are uncomfortable with such events. Schonfeld et al. (1994) noted:

> As schools face an escalating number of crises, the probability that any child or group of children will experience violence or sudden death of a friend and/or loved one is increasing. These events often require a response from the school in order to address the children's developmental needs during times of crisis and uncertainty. These crisis periods can disrupt learning, at a minimum, and also have the potential to retard children's emotional and psychological adjustment to the event and impair their subsequent development. . . . Crises that affect students will also have a significant impact on the staff and the school as a whole [p. 156].

Also, as Deaton and Berkan (1995) recently observed, when school staff decide not to guide students to an understanding of a death, "an opportunity is lost to prepare students for the reality of life and death in an atmosphere where the normal grief reaction can be dealt with in a safe, supportive climate" (p. 113).

TRAUMA-INDUCED PSYCHOLOGICAL DISEQUILIBRIUM

When a child or adolescent dies by suicide, the emotional impact is felt throughout the school the youth attended, the entire school district, and often the whole community (Bozigar et al., 1993; Celotta, 1995; Sandoval and Brock, 1996). Cleiren and Diekstra (1995) recently made the following observations:

> One basic survival quality is our ability to organize our world, both on the outside by moving about, and influencing it with our actions, and internally by organizing the information coming to us through our senses into meaningful "schemas." What we literally do is "make sense" of our life: we ascribe meaning to what is happening to us, so that we, on the basis of this knowledge, steer ourselves through the seas and storms toward our goal with

as little damage as possible. In our life, we learn, build up a more and more differentiated image of the world, including abilities, skills, conceptions of "how things work", "what is important", and also *who* is important [pp. 19–20].

This set of beliefs and cognitive processes has been termed the *assumptive world* by Parkes (1988), and bereavement as a consequence of the death of a young person by suicide is likely to upset many of individual survivors' assumptions. For all of the people (e.g., peers, family members, teachers, administrators), left in the aftermath of a student's suicide, the death "breaks the barrier of complacency and resistance in [their] assumptive worlds" and induces "a profound psychological crisis" (Janoff-Bulman, 1992, p. 61). This shattering of assumptions caused by the trauma of a suicidal death of a young person creates a psychological disequilibrium in the survivors (Janoff-Bulman, 1992). Postvention assistance must provide an opportunity for survivors to address this psychological disequilibrium (Carter and Brooks, 1990, 1991; Dunne, 1992; Valente and Saunders, 1993; Mauk and Rodgers, 1994).

Young people who experience the death of a peer by suicide are in crisis (Mauk and Rodgers, 1994). The suicide of a youth is a particularly psychologically malignant mode of death for friends and acquaintances who are left behind—the "survivors." For the child or adolescent survivor, who views the self as indestructible, the death of a friend or acquaintance challenges his or her ability to cope. Recognition of the special features of this type of loss is vital to understanding the emotional and behavioral responses that are common to peer survivors of an adolescent's suicide (see Figure 1).

PROVISION OF POSTVENTION SERVICES FOR SURVIVORS

Carter and Brooks (1990), the American Association of Suicidology (1997), Mauk and Weber (1991), Mauk and Rodgers (1994), Renaud (1995), and others have noted the need for proactive and appropriate postvention activities directed at peers left behind in the aftermaths of such tragedies. Postvention work, as a proactive response of a caring institution to the needs of its members, the students and staff, is an

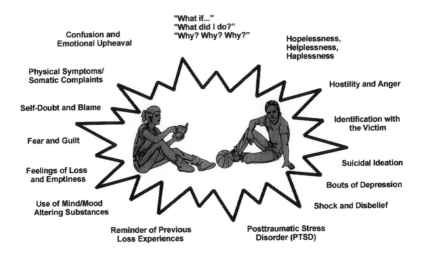

Confusion and
Emotional Upheaval

"What if..."
"What did I do?"
"Why? Why? Why?"

Hopelessness,
Helplessness,
Haplessness

Physical Symptoms/
Somatic Complaints

Self-Doubt and Blame

Fear and Guilt

Feelings of Loss
and Emptiness

Use of Mind/Mood
Altering Substances

Hostility and Anger

Identification with
the Victim

Suicidal Ideation

Bouts of Depression

Shock and Disbelief

Reminder of Previous
Loss Experiences

Posttraumatic Stress
Disorder (PTSD)

Figure 1 Examples of potential effects of a youth's suicide on surviving peers (From Mauk and Rodgers, 1994, p. 110). Adapted by permission.

opportunity gained in the face of crisis (Carter and Brooks, 1990; Mauk and Rodgers, 1994; McEvoy and McEvoy, 1994).

Postvention is a form of tertiary prevention and refers to efforts made to address the painful effects on individuals affected to varying degrees by a traumatic event or crisis. With particular reference to suicide, postvention is (a) the process, after a suicide, during which an individual and/or a family works toward emotional and psychological recovery and readjustment to a healthy lifestyle and (b) the provision of interventions combining education and counseling to prevent bereavement complications for individuals left behind in the wake of the suicide (Hatton, 1977; Carter and Brooks, 1990, 1991; Philip, 1990; Valente and Saunders, 1993; Sandoval and Brock, 1996).

Some experts have argued that the most important purpose of postvention is the prevention of imitative suicidal behavior (contagion) among peers (Hazell, 1991; Bozigar et al., 1993). Other professionals have asserted that the primary task of postvention is resolution of grief in the survivors (Poland, 1989). However, the prevention of suicidal contagion need not be sacrificed for the task of assisting with grief resolution among survivors (Capuzzi, 1994). For example, Carter and Brooks (1991) stated that, although the immediate goal of postvention is diffusion of the toxic effects of the suicide and prevention of further

184

suicidal activity among the surviving peers, additional objectives are repairing of damaged support systems and accessing previously unused internal, interpersonal, and professional resources (American Association of Suicidology, 1997; Tedeschi and Calhoun, 1993).

In fact, Brent et al. (1992), in their study of the effects of exposure to suicide among the friends and acquaintances of adolescent suicide victims, reported that the current emphasis of school-based suicide postvention activities for the prevention of imitative suicide may be mismatched to the needs of peer survivors, who frequently manifest severe, long-term depressive symptomatology. Thus, it appears that an equally yoked, two-pronged approach to suicide postvention (prevention of contagion and grief resolution) must be undertaken by schools and community agencies.

Involvement of the School in Postvention Efforts

RATIONALE FOR SCHOOL-BASED POSTVENTION SERVICES

The school is a critical force in suicide postvention efforts with youth. Because children and adolescents spend many hours of each week in the school setting, it is a crucial and logical site for implementation of a suicide postvention program. Contemporary schools are expected to address not only the intellectual needs of students but also students' emotional, social, and physical needs (Petersen and Straub, 1992; Turner, 1996).

Smith and Garza (1989) cited three considerations that justify the school's involvement in postvention activities for peer survivors after the suicide of an adolescent: (a) Schools have the responsibility of helping adolescents develop into productive citizens who can contribute positively to society, (b) schools have the responsibility to identify and attempt to identify and resolve problems that interfere with the educational process, and (c) schools have the opportunity and resources to identify and offer assistance to at-risk adolescents. Likewise, Pynoos and Nader (1990) observed that the school is the optimal site for postvention following a disaster or other trauma because (a) it is most convenient to children and their families and (b) the stigmatization that accompanies use of mental health agencies is skirted. They asserted,

"The school is an ideal locus to involve parents, teachers, and children in preventively oriented trauma response programs" (p. 228).

A caring, positive environment, personal attachments, and affable involvements among students and staff in contemporary schools contribute substantially to what distinguishes excellent schools (Pitcher and Poland, 1992). However, it is this same environment and affective quality of student–staff relationships that shocks and emotionally devastates school administrators, faculty, and staff when a student in their care commits suicide. Consequently, Pitcher and Poland (1992) observed that, without appropriate preparation, training, and understanding, the crisis of a student's suicide can interfere significantly with the ability of school administrators, teachers, and other staff to function competently and to address their own and surviving students' needs. Thus, when a student takes his or her life, a logical place to provide postvention services is the school that the deceased attended, because many of the decedent's peers (and staff who knew them) will be affected by the death (Mattison and Spirito, 1993; Mauk and Rodgers, 1994; Mackesy-Amiti et al., 1996).

ASSESSING THE IMPACT OF THE DEATH ON THE SCHOOL COMMUNITY

Komar (1994) made the following observations with respect to school crises: (a) There is an ostensible connection between the cause of the unexpected death (e.g., homicide, suicide, accident) and the nature of the student response, (b) a key indicator of the magnitude of stress to be manifested by the school population is the popularity of the individual(s) who died, and (c) the response of school administrators and key faculty members can have a substantial impact on the severity of the repercussions that a given school will experience as a result of the death.

Brock, Sandoval, and Lewis (1996, p. 85) have advised school administrators, staff, and community mental health professionals to consider the following aspects and questions when they are gauging the impact of a crisis on their school and community:

1. *The popularity of the victim.* If the victim was popular or well-known, a more substantial impact can be expected in the school/community.

2. *Individuals' exposure to or involvement in the crisis.* The greater the exposure or involvement in the crisis, the greater the impact of the crisis will be for individuals. For example, a tragic incident on school grounds would be likely to affect the entire student body, whereas a crisis event that occurred far away from the school that involved only a few students would have a less severe effect.

3. *History of similar crises.* If similar crises have happened to the school in the past, the current crisis may likely rekindle old crisis reactions in addition to generating a new trauma. Thus, a more substantial reaction to the current crisis may result.

4. *Recency of other crises.* If other crises have happened to the school recently, students' and staff members' resiliency may be reduced, and more substantial crisis reactions may result. If no recent crises have happened, a less dramatic impact might be expected.

5. *Available resources.* If few personal, family, school, and community resources are available to help students and staff cope with the crisis, more substantial crisis reactions may occur.

6. *Timing of the crisis event.* If the crisis occurred during a vacation or early during a weekend, its impact on the school may be less than if the crisis occurred while school was in session. In this case, it is possible that students will have dealt with the crisis away from school—on their own or with their families. Also, rumors are generally spread more quickly when children and adolescents are congregating in groups at school. Finally, when a crisis occurs during a vacation, the school has more time to prepare and thus is able to respond to students' and staff members' needs and reactions more effectively.

IDENTIFICATION OF "AT-RISK" SURVIVORS

Although everyone who is exposed to suicide requires some level of care and will try to understand the suicide in his or her own way, not all students are equally affected by the suicide of a peer. Some students are at greater personal risk (Catone and Schatz, 1991; Blau, 1996; Sandoval and Brock, 1996). Cleiren and Diekstra (1995) made the following observations:

It is especially important to recognize that those bereaved who suffer a combination of a substantial loss, little material resources, weak personal and social skills, and little belief in their own abilities to deal with it, are a risk group. They tend to isolate from others and the fabric of their social and personal life tears further, making them suffer, in fact, more and more losses [p. 34].

Thus, those young people who have particular psychological and social vulnerability may become dangerously at-risk as they collide with the experience of suicide (Hazell, 1991). For example, Ruof, Harris, and Robbie (1987) and Ruof and Harris (1988) have described several types of young people who become a greater risk after a suicide. These include:

1. Any young person who participated in any way with the completed suicide, helped write the suicide note, was mentioned in the note, provided the means, or was involved with a "suicide pact."
2. Any young person who knew of the suicide plans and did not tell anyone.
3. Any young person who is a sibling, other relative, or best friend of the deceased youth.
4. Any young people who were self-appointed therapists to the deceased youth and who had made it their responsibility to keep the person's problems and plans a secret.
5. Any young person with a history of suicidal threats and attempts himself or herself.
6. Any young person who identified with the victim's situation.
7. Any young person who had reason to feel guilty about things that he or she said or did to the student before the student's death.
8. Any young person who did not take a suicide threat seriously, had been too busy to talk with a suicide victim who asked for help, and/or observed events that they later learned were indicative of the victim's suicidal intent.
9. Any young person who had recently punished or threatened to punish the victim for some misdeed.
10. Other young people desperate for any reason who now see suicide as a viable alternative.

Hazell and Lewin (1993a, b), in their research with peer survivors of adolescent suicide attempters and completers, found that friends of both suicide attempters and completers show a greater degree of disturbance than comparison groups. Hazell and Lewin observed that interventions could be directed usefully to friends of suicide attempters both in the context of exposure to completed suicide and in response to exposure to attempted suicide. Additionally, Martin, Kuller, and Hazell (1992) found that adolescents with depression, recent thoughts of killing themselves, and admitted episodes of recent self-harm were more likely to know of a suicide, and the suicide of a peer may hold more meaning for them in terms of confirming their beliefs about suicide, making them more prone to imitating the peer. Martin et al. concluded that "it is toward identification of this vulnerable group that preventive efforts should be aimed following an adolescent suicide" (p. 23).

Time-Limited and Long-Term Postvention Processes

THE IMMEDIATE RESPONSE
AND PSYCHOLOGICAL FIRST AID

As with any crisis situation, the hallmarks of effective postvention efforts are immediacy and flexibility of response (Grossman et al., 1995) as well as empathy, warmth, and genuineness on the part of any interveners (Hendricks and McKean, 1995). Postvention activities provided immediately after the suicide might be considered "psychological first aid" (Slaikeu, 1990, p. 102). *Psychological first aid* (a) is provided immediately, (b) lasts minutes or hours, (c) is provided by counselors, school-based psychologists, teachers, administrators, nurses, and so forth, (d) is provided in the immediate school community, and (e) has as its goals the reestablishment of immediate coping, provision of support, reduction of lethality, and linking of affected students and educators to helping resources (Slaikeu, 1990; Brock et al., 1996).

How the school reacts in the immediate situation of a student's suicide as well as in the aftermath and ensuing recovery period may substantially affect individual young people's recovery. Adequate postvention at the school level should include (a) appropriate information sharing and discussion with relevant groups of students within the school, (b) screening of individuals at high risk, and (c) triage of carefully identified students into appropriate treatment (Davidson, 1990). Researchers conducting longitudinal studies of bereavement have shown that there generally is a quick recovery of mental health and a decrease of complaints related to bereavement during the first year with relatively little change occurring after this period (Cleiren and Diekstra, 1995). Also, it appears that individuals who are initially effective in coping with the loss remain effective as time passes (Cleiren, 1993).

SHORT-TERM INDIVIDUAL AND GROUP WORK WITH SURVIVORS

The trauma of the suicide of a peer and/or friend may make it difficult for child and adolescent survivors to reach out for support as they become overwhelmed by feelings of abandonment, rejection, social isolation, and confusion. Yet, many of them may not be able to cope alone with the resultant psychological and social disequilibrium created by the tragic event and trauma of the suicide. Individual counseling can provide a safe place for sharing grief, confusion, anger, or fear (Mauk and Weber, 1991). For some youth survivors, individual therapy is most effective because they relate best to one trusted person. For other youth survivors, a support group of similar survivors facilitated by a school psychologist, school counselor, or other mental health professional knowledgeable about suicide and bereavement is effective (Battle, 1984; Catone and Schatz, 1991; Tedeschi and Calhoun, 1993).

Participation in therapeutic group work is considered by some professionals to be "the treatment of choice because it creates community, puts the locus of control on the individual, and emphasizes interaction and growth—all essential ingredients in bereavement work" (Zimpfer, 1991, p. 47). The broad purposes of dedicated therapeutic groups are to (a) increase people's knowledge of themselves and others, (b) assist people to clarify the changes they most want to make in their own life, and (c) give people some of the tools necessary to make those desired changes (Corey and Corey, 1987).

Therapeutic group work provides a safe setting in which "to try these changes on for size as well" (Moore and Freeman, 1995, p. 43). Freeman (1991) wrote:

Group counseling can be an appropriate vehicle through which to facilitate the survivors' search for understanding and resolution. . . . The goals of a group counseling approach are to facilitate movement through the stages of the grief process by providing a supportive environment in which those directly affected by a suicide can progress. Participants are encouraged to express their needs in dealing with their grief and also to set goals as to what they would like to accomplish in the group [p. 328].

Perhaps the most pressing need of youth survivors in the therapeutic group setting is normalization of their complex reactions to the suicidal death (Wrobleski, 1984). The group provides a safe environment in which the expression of complex emotions following the suicidal death of a peer, so often discouraged or prevented in the community, becomes the rule and not the exception for the survivors (Battle, 1984; Schwab, 1986). Moore and Freeman (1995) observed that sharing common feelings and experiences is instrumental in the acceptance of survivors' own (as well as community members') reactions to the death. Yet, "the very stigma attached to suicidal death can prevent survivors from joining groups specifically formed to address this and other issues that they face" (Moore and Freeman, 1995, p. 44). Thus, Wrobleski (1984) advocated for a support group, rather than a therapy group, for suicide survivors, "because bereavement is a normal process following any type of death" (Moore and Freeman, 1995, p. 45). Similarly, Tedeschi and Calhoun (1993) noted that, as a consequence of finding a common human bond with other individuals who are bereaved, "people leaving bereavement support groups often speak of a greater feeling of closeness with family and friends, and a new or deeper understanding of the universality of human experience" (p. 52). Morganett (1990, pp. 181–202) has provided some excellent guidance for educators seeking to design and implement groups for young people who are struggling to cope with grief or loss.

FOLLOW-UP SERVICES FOR SURVIVORS

Although postvention is an activity that should focus on doing what is necessary to control the school environment yet process the emotional turmoil of the survivors in the "here and now," another component of postvention is the provision of long-term follow-up services to affected survivors. Postvention assistance that extends well beyond mitigating the immediate impact of the suicide for significantly affected students and staff might be termed *crisis therapy* (Slaikeu, 1990, p. 102). Crisis therapy (a) is provided when the individual is unable to work through crises on his or her own, (b) lasts weeks or months, (c) is provided by school and community mental health professionals, (d) is provided in school and community counseling settings, and (e) has as its goals the resolution of the crisis, working through the crisis event, integration of the event into the fabric of life, and establishment of openness and readiness to face the future (Slaikeu, 1990; Catone and Schatz, 1991; Celotta, 1995; Brock et al., 1996).

The recent findings of Brent et al. (1993) have supported the notion that, although an immediate, short-term, triage-centered postvention response is necessary, it may indeed not be enough. Brent et al. made the following observations:

> It appears that there is a mismatch between the brief, intensive, time-limited interventions of postvention, and the needs of members of the social networks of suicide victims, who seem to frequently experience long, debilitating depressive disorders. Therefore, more intensive clinical follow-up for friends of suicide victims is recommended; and the clinician should be careful not to dismiss depressive symptomatology too quickly as attributable to "normal grief" [p. 516].

With regard to peer survivors of a youth's suicide, for some students, "a protracted grief- and stress-related symptomatology characterized by intrusive thoughts and images triggering avoidant defenses persists over weeks" (Kaltreider, 1990, p. 202). Thus, a less intensive, long-term follow-up program provided by a crisis intervention team is a necessary complement to the initial postvention response. The program should be directed toward the daily living with the loss and grief over a year or more following the student's death and should address, usually through referral to appropriate community agencies, manifestations of psychological morbidity (e.g., new-onset depression, substance abuse) as a result of complications of bereavement. Fortunately, however, Cleiren and Diekstra (1995) have observed that

> the violence or abruptness of suicide as a form of death does not predestine the prospects of recovery in the bereaved. The fact

that most bereaved are capable of making a difference by using and rebuilding resources, and applying adequate adaptational strategies, outlines both the goal and the basis for therapeutic interventions in suicide bereavement [p. 34].

Although surviving students are empowered by an effective postvention response, they are not the only beneficiaries. Administration and staff can also be empowered by learning valuable lessons in the aftermath of such a trauma—lessons that may serve them well in dealing with future crises. Zinner (1987) observed:

Individual students gain much insight and understanding when they partake in the group's response to the loss of a friend or co-student. But students graduate, taking their newly acquired knowledge with them. It is the school faculty and staff who must be willing and able to facilitate group survivorship responses. Only they can gain the experience and perspective on what helps a group survive and benefit from a member's death [p. 501].

"NON-IDEAL" VERSUS "IDEAL" POSTVENTIONS

Komar (1994) observed that the main cause for non-ideal conditions for postvention work in a school is the underestimation by the school community of the extent of the repercussions that are incident to an untimely death such as the suicide of a student. The most common preventable non-ideal postvention conditions include (a) no existing internal crisis maintenance structures, (b) no preparations have been made for incorporation of outside resources, (c) haphazard and harried communication of facts, (d) basic school structure not followed (i.e., maintaining the regular class schedule), (e) teachers and other staff not given the physical, emotional, or informational support to cope with the extent of grief exhibited, and (f) political or "turf" issues preventing productive coexistence of resources (Komar, 1994, p. 39). Accordingly, nonpreventable postvention conditions are those that are created by (a) repercussions to the death that far exceed the capabilities of all of the combined, available resources and (b) basic facts of the death either unavailable and/or altered due to constraints on confidentiality (Komar, 1994, p. 40).

In contrast, in the ideal postvention case, the school (a) will have a postvention policy in place before a crisis or tragedy and (b) will have structured its own crisis management resources as well as planned for the inclusion of outside consultation with and assistance from community mental health professionals (Dunne-Maxim et al., 1992; Schonfeld, 1993; Hundley and Bratton, 1994; Komar, 1994; Mauk, Gibson, and Rodgers, 1994; Mauk and Rodgers, 1994; Schonfeld et al., 1994; Celotta, 1995; Roberts, 1995). Komar (1994) asserted that there are two fundamental components to the helping process of postvention after a severe crisis and traumatic event in and around a school: "pre-existing crisis management or student support teams in the school" (p. 44) and "the availability of a postvention team who can flood a school with highly trained professionals in the area of grief counseling and lethality assessment" (p. 44). Gleaned from the literature reviewed up to this point, some general guidelines for proactive suicide postvention in school settings appear in Table 1; in Table 2, we list selected resources for developing and implementing school-based crisis response plans and postcrisis grief interventions.

THE SCHOOL'S RESPONSE
IN A COMMUNITY FRAMEWORK

Grossman et al. (1995) have asserted, "A student's sudden death by suicide is one of the most difficult crises confronting communities" (p. 18). The Centers for Disease Control (1988) have recommended that an idiosyncratic community plan be implemented "when a potentially traumatic death occurs in the community—especially if the person who dies is an adolescent" (p. 6) to aid both in personal adjustment of surviving peers and others and to address possible contagion effects (Wenckstern and Leenaars, 1993). In this regard, a community-school network is an effective strategy for planning and implementing a postsuicide response for surviving peers (Mauk and Rodgers, 1994). Hicks (1990) has described such a network:

> A postvention network of support is *community involvement* to deal with the tragedy of youth suicide. . . . The task of a community postvention support mechanism is to develop a responsive support mechanism for survivors of an adolescent suicide

TABLE 1

Ten Guidelines for Proactive Suicide Postvention in Schools

1. There is no substitute for planning. A school should have a policy, plan, and implementation process in place before a suicide occurs. Ideally, a school and/or school district should have a team of professionals managed by a designated postvention coordinator.
2. Workshops on reactions to trauma, crisis management, and postvention procedures should be conducted by school psychologists, school counselors, and community mental health professionals for school administrators, teachers, and other staff.
3. Recognize that, although there are common elements, each suicide situation has unique aspects and, thus, must be managed accordingly.
4. The school administrator or principal should contact the faculty and staff and apprise them of the suicide and the postvention plans and convene a meeting of faculty and staff within the school as soon as possible.
5. Simultaneously, the postvention coordinator should be contacted, and he or she should contact, brief, and mobilize the postvention team.
6. The students in the school should be notified of the facts of the suicide death directly and as early as possible, ideally by teachers in individual classes.
7. A school-based spokesperson should be assigned to deal with the media immediately after the suicide has been confirmed. Highlight and emphasize the positive activities and procedures being conducted by the school in the aftermath of the tragedy.
8. Locations should be assigned within the school community at which (a) psychological triage of affected students and school staff can be conducted to refer students and staff members to appropriate care settings and services, (b) screening of individuals at "high risk" can be done, and (c) psychological first aid can be provided.
9. A letter should be sent to all parents (a) to inform them of the facts of the situation, (b) to apprise them of the actions taken by the school and how to contact the school for further information, and (c) to alert them to possible reactions of their child/adolescent to the trauma of the suicide.
10. Arrange for long-term therapeutic and educational follow-up with students and staff through workshops and linkages of existing school resources with community mental health professionals and consultants.

---

event. . . . The concern of postvention is for the emotional health of the students, their parents and the school faculty [pp. 80, 81, 86].

Because suicide crises can and often do affect social systems larger than educational systems, school-community linkages extend far beyond mere identification of students, and staff in need of postvention assistance; such linkages must ethically include individually and organizationally responsive intervention components too (Philip, 1990; American Association of Suicidology, 1997; Dunne-Maxim et al., 1992; Adelman, 1993; Schonfeld, 1993; Schonfeld et al., 1994; Paul, 1995; Richardson, 1995; Roberts, 1995; Mackesy-Amiti et al., 1996). As Schonfeld (1993) wrote:

TABLE 2

TWELVE CRISIS INTERVENTION AND DEATH POSTVENTION RESOURCES FOR SCHOOLS

1. Adams, D. W. & Deveau, E. J., (ed.) (1995), *Beyond the Innocence of Childhood: Vol. 3—Helping Children and Adolescents Cope with Death and Bereavement*. Amityville, NY: Baywood.
2. Bozigar, J. A., Brent, D. A., Hindmarsh, K., Kerr, M. M., McQuiston, L. & Turich, C. (1993), *Postvention Standards Manual: A Guide for a School's Response in the Aftermath of a Suicide*. Pittsburgh: University of Pittsburgh Medical Center, Western Psychiatric Institute and Clinic, Services for Teenagers at Risk.
3. Brock, S. E., Sandoval, J. & Lewis, S. (1996), *Preparing for Crises in the Schools: A Manual for Building School Crisis Response Teams*. Brandon, VT: Clinical Psychology.
4. Corr, C. A. & Balk, D. E., (ed.) (1996), *Handbook of Adolescent Death and Bereavement*. New York: Springer.
5. Corr, C. A. & Corr, D. M., (ed.) (1996), *Handbook of Childhood Death and Bereavement*. New York: Springer.
6. Deaton, R. L. & Berkan, W. A. (1995), *Planning and Managing Death Issues in the Schools*. Westport, CT: Greenwood.
7. Johnson, K. (1993), *School Crisis Management*. Alameda, CA: Hunter House.
8. Oates, M. D. (1993), *Death in the School Community: A Handbook for Counselors, Teachers, and Administrators*. Alexandria, VA: American Association for Counseling & Development.
9. Petersen, S. & Straub, R. L. (1992), *School Crisis Survival Guide: Management Techniques and Materials for Counselors and Administrators*. West Nyack, NY: Center for Applied Research in Education.
10. Pitcher, G. D. & Poland, S. (1992), *Crisis Intervention in the Schools*. New York: Guilford.
11. Steele, W. (1992), *Preventing Self-Destruction: A Manual for School Crisis Response Teams*. Holmes Beach, FL: Learning Publications.
12. Van Ornum, W. & Mordock, J. B. (1990), *Crisis Counseling with Children and Adolescents: A Guide for Nonprofessional Counselors*. New York: Continuum.

School staff should have contingency plans and preestablished liaisons with community resources that will allow expedited referrals for counseling services that are either inappropriate for school-based intervention or that are unavailable in the school. . . . Identification of problems, without the capacity for intervention, is a disservice to the students and staff [p. 657].

Therefore, it is important that postvention plans extend from the school to the community, with both contributing requisite resources through established communication and staff allocation liaisons and networks (Hazell, 1991; Dunne-Maxim et al., 1992; Adelman, 1993; Hundley and Bratton, 1994; Mauk and Rodgers, 1994; Roberts, 1995; Mackesy-Amiti et al., 1996; Sandoval and Brock, 1996). Schonfeld et al. (1994) noted that "planning how to respond to a crisis can be both an enabling and empowering process and need not represent an incremental crisis" (p. 165). Hicks (1990) has stated:

As each community develops a network of awareness, education, and action—a network of educators, parents, and youth—this network will translate into a system of caring and responsiveness for at-risk youth. This system of support will communicate understanding and concern and be a comprehensive and effective preventive mechanism [p. 10].

Suicide Postvention Roles for Psychiatrists in the Schools

Psychiatrists are key mental health resources in many communities. As such, they can participate in many ways in the planning and provision of efficacious suicide postvention in schools and their communities at large, including but not limited to the following (Klingman and Ben-Eli, 1981; Peck and Berkovitz, 1987; Brent et al., 1988; Brent et al., 1989; Trachta, 1988; Klingman, 1989; Davidson, 1990; Blom et al., 1991; Lamb et al., 1991; Mattison, 1993a, b; Mattison and Spirito, 1993; Hundley and Bratton, 1994; Schonfeld et al., 1994; Grossman et al., 1995; Hendricks and McKean, 1995; Paul, 1995; Mackesy-Amiti et al., 1996): (a) participation in the development of an organizational/community model for crisis intervention, (b) training professionals and paraprofessionals in crisis intervention theory, process, and applications to school-based suicide postvention activities, (c) assessment of a school's and community's readiness to respond and actual response to a crisis such as a parasuicide or completed suicide, (d) on-site psychological screening of student/staff who were exposed to a suicidal event, (e) providing on-site postvention consultation and follow-up services, (f) referral of students/staff in need of long-term postvention assistance, and (g) psychological autopsies of suicide completers. Trachta (1988), in his description of the involvement of the staff of a psychiatric hospital in postvention efforts in school systems, made the following observations regarding schools:

[Schools] are performing functions that family service agencies used to perform, as well as functions that were once performed by families. *Those of us in the hospital setting are in an ideal situation to teach them the various things they can do and how to adapt techniques to their own systems. . . .* Schools need ways to handle catastrophic events surrounding the death of a student. *Postvention should actively provide the school with a meaningful response to trauma that seems to help school personnel feel better informed and able to handle future traumatic events* [pp. 167–168, italics added].

Psychiatrists must make themselves known and available to school systems and, in collaboration with school-based mental health professionals (e.g., school counselors, school social workers, school psychologists), must take a proactive role in the development and support of suicide postvention strategies in schools and communities.

SUMMARY

Unfortunately, each year in the United States more than 5,000 young people between the ages of 5 and 24 take their own lives. Poland (1995) recently observed that "schools are frequently not prepared to deal with the aftermath of a suicide yet few events are more disruptive" (p. 464). Thus, schools and their staffs must not only prepare for the administrative disruption to a school as a result of a student's suicide, but they must also be ready to provide postvention assistance to the children and adolescents who are the friends and acquaintances of the deceased and who are left behind in the tragic wake of the suicide event. Deaton and Berkan (1995) noted that a review of the first-person-account literature on survivors left behind in the wake of a friend's suicide reveals the unjustified guilt and the pain they endure until they move through the individualistic and discontinuous grief process. Deaton and Berkan further observed:

It is the grief process that allows survivors to find their own answers to a friend's death . . . As time passes, students will find some answers that will be comforting for them and they will discover that it is possible to eventually accept the fact that we do not have all the answers about why certain deaths occur [p. 122].

Also, it is critical to note that the suicide of an adolescent is simultaneously a time of crisis and a time of opportunity for a school and for the students caught up in the tragic aftermath of a young person's suicide. At its heart, postvention is an opportunistic process of assisting survivors in building bridges over the troubled waters created in the wake of a peer's suicide (Mauk and Rodgers, 1994). Wenckstern and Leenaars (1993) recently made the following observations with respect to traumatic events and schools:

Schools are not normally equipped to address the mental health needs and possible post-traumatic stress reactions in many survivors after traumas such as suicide, homicide, serious accidents, or hostage taking. School postvention programs that utilize a team approach have an important role in our schools and school communities to assist survivors by fostering positive adjustment strategies, forestalling possible long-term psychological damage as well as addressing possible imitative/contagion effects [p. 169].

Thus, with planned and appropriate postvention assistance from a team of caring adults in the school setting and involvement of professionals from community mental health agencies, children and adolescents who remain behind as survivors in the wake of a student's suicide can be sustained through the psychosocial trauma of the death.

REFERENCES

Adelman, H. S. (1993), School-linked mental health interventions: Toward mechanisms for service coordination and integration. *J. Comm. Psychol.*, 21:309–319.

American Association of Suicidology (1997), *Suicide Postvention Guidelines*, 2nd ed. Washington, DC: American Association of Suicidology.

Anderson, R. N., Kochanek, K. D. & Murphy, S. L. (1997). Report of final mortality statistics, 1995. *Monthly Vital Statistics Report,* 45(11, Suppl. 2), 1–80. (This report is available from the Centers for Disease Control and Prevention, National Center for Health Statistics, Hyattsville, MD 20782.)

Battle, A. O. (1984), Group therapy for survivors of suicide. *Crisis,* 5:45–58.

Berman, A. L. & Jobes, D. A. (1991), *Adolescent Suicide: Assessment and Intervention*. Washington, DC: American Psychological Association.

Blau, G. M. (1996), Adolescent suicide and depression. In: *Adolescent Dysfunctional Behavior: Causes, Interventions, and Prevention*, ed. G. M. Blau & T. P. Gullotta. Thousand Oaks, CA: Sage, pp. 187–205.

Blom, G. E., Etkind, S. L. & Carr, W. J. (1991), Psychological interventions after child and adolescent disasters in the community. *Child Psychiatr. & Human Devel.*, 21:257–266.

Bozigar, J. A., Brent, D. A., Hindmarsh, K., Kerr, M. M., McQuiston, L. & Turich, C. (1993), *Postvention Standards Manual*. Pittsburgh: University of Pittsburgh Medical Center, Western Psychiatric Institute and Clinic, Services for Teenagers at Risk (STAR Center).

Brent, D. A., Kerr, M. M., Goldstein, C., Bozigar, J., Wartella, M. & Allan, M. J. (1989), *J. Amer. Acad. Child & Adoles. Psychiat.*, 28:918–924.

———— Perper, J. A., Kolko, D. J. & Zelenak, J. P. (1988), The psychological autopsy:Methodological considerations for the study of adolescent suicide. *J. Amer. Acad. Child & Adoles. Psychiat.*, 27:362–366.

———— ———— Moritz, G., Allman, C., Friend, A., Schweers, J., Roth, C., Balach, L. & Harrington, K. (1992), Psychiatric effects of exposure to suicide among the friends and acquaintances of adolescent suicide victims. *J. Amer. Acad. Child & Adoles. Psychiat.*, 31:629–640.

———— ———— ———— ———— Schweers, J., Roth, C., Balach, L., Cannobio & Liotus, L. (1993), Psychiatric sequelae to the loss of an adolescent peer to suicide. *J. Amer. Acad. Child & Adoles. Psychiat.*, 32:509–517.

Brock, S. E., Sandoval, J. & Lewis, S. (1996), *Preparing for Crises in the Schools*. Brandon, VT: Clinical Psychology.

Capuzzi, D. (1994), *Suicide Prevention in the Schools*. Alexandria, VA: American Counseling Association.

Carter, B. F. & Brooks, A. (1990), Suicide postvention: Crisis or opportunity? *School Counselor*, 37:378–390.

———— ———— (1991), Child and adolescent survivors of suicide. In: *Life Span Perspectives of Suicide*, ed. A. A. Leenaars. New York: Plenum, pp. 231–258.

Catone, W. V. & Schatz, M. T. (1991), The crisis moment: A school's response to the event of a suicide. *School Psychol. Internat.*, 12:17–23.

Celotta, B. (1995), The aftermath of suicide: Postvention in a school setting. *J. Mental Health Counsel.*, 17:397–412.

Centers for Disease Control (1988), Recommendations for a community plan for the prevention and containment of suicide clusters. *Morbidity & Mortality Wkly. Rep.*, 37(Suppl. S-6):1–11.

Cimbolic, P. & Jobes, D. A. (1990), *Youth Suicide: Issues.* Springfield, IL: Thomas.

Cleiren, M. P. H. D. (1993), *Bereavement and Adaptation.* Washington, DC: Hemisphere.

———— & Diekstra, R. F. W. (1995), After the loss: Bereavement after suicide and other types of death. In: *The Impact of Suicide*, ed. B. L. Mishara. New York: Springer, pp. 7–39.

Corey, M. S. & Corey, G. (1987), *Groups: Process and Practice.* Pacific Grove, CA: Brooks/Cole.

Davidson, S. (1990), Management. In: *Suicide in Children and Adolescents*, ed. G. MacLean. Lewiston, NY: Hogrefe & Huber, pp. 89–127.

Deaton, R. L. & Berkan, W. A. (1995), *Planning and Managing Death Issues in the Schools.* Westport, CT: Greenwood.

Doka, K. J. (1989), Disenfranchised grief. In: *Disenfranchised Grief*, ed. K. J. Doka. Lexington, MA: Heath, pp. 3–11.

Dunn, R. G. & Morrish-Vidners, D. (1987–1988), The psychological and social experience of suicide survivors. *Omega: J. Death & Dying*, 18:175-215.

Dunne, E. J. (1992), Psychoeducational intervention strategies for survivors of suicide. *Crisis*, 13(1):35–40.

Dunne-Maxim, K., Godin, S., Lamb, F., Sutton, C. & Underwood, M. (1992), The aftermath of youth suicide—Providing postvention services for the school and community. *Crisis*, 13(1):16–22.

Freeman, S. J. (1991), Group facilitation of the grieving process with those bereaved by suicide. *J. Counsel. & Devel.*, 69:328–331.

Glass, J. C. (1991), Death, loss, and grief among middle school children: Implications for the school counselor. *Element. School Guid. & Counsel.*, 26:139–148.

Grossman, J., Hirsch, J., Goldenberg, D., Libby, S., Fendrich, M., Mackesy-Amiti, M. E., Mazur, C. & Chance, G. H. (1995), Strategies for school-based response to loss: Proactive training and postvention consultation. *Crisis*, 16(1):18–26.

Hatton, C. (1977), *Suicide: Assessment and Intervention.* New York: Appleton–Century–Crofts.

Hazell, P. (1991), Postvention after teenage suicide: An Australian experience. *J. Adoles.*, 14:335–342.

———— & Lewin, T. (1993a), An evaluation of postvention following adolescent suicide. *Suicide & Life-Threatening Behav.*, 23:101–109.

———— ———— (1993b), Friends of adolescent suicide attempters and completers. *J. Amer. Acad. Child & Adoles. Psychiat.*, 32:76–81.

Hendricks, J. E. & McKean, J. B. (1995), *Crisis Intervention.* Springfield, IL: Thomas.

Hicks, B. B. (1990), *Youth Suicide.* Bloomington, IN: National Educational Service.

Hundley, M. & Bratton, S. (1994), Adolescent loss and the school community: Don't let them slip through your fingers. *Texas Counsel. Assn. J.*, 22:10–22.

James, J. W. & Cherry, F. (1988), *The Grief Recovery Handbook.* New York: Harper & Row.

Janoff-Bulman, R. (1992), *Shattered Assumptions.* New York: Lexington Books.

Kaltreider, N. B. (1990), The impact of a medical student's suicide. *Suicide and Life-Threatening Behav.*, 20:195–205.

Kliman, A. S. (1978), *Crisis: Psychological Aid for Recovery and Growth.* New York: Holt, Rinehart & Winston.

Klingman, A. (1989), School-based emergency intervention following an adolescent's suicide. *Death Studies*, 13:263–274.

———— & Ben-Eli, Z. (1981), A school community in disaster: Primary and secondary prevention in situational crises. *Profess. Psychol.*, 12:523–533.

Komar, A. A. (1994), Adolescent school crises: Structures, issues, and techniques for postventions. *Internat. J. Adoles. & Youth*, 5:35–46.

Lamb, F., Dunne-Maxim, K., Underwood, M. & Sutton, C. (1991), Postvention from the viewpoint of consultants. In: *Suicide Prevention in Schools*, ed. A. A. Leenaars & S. Wenckstern. New York: Hemisphere, pp. 213–227.

Mackesy-Amiti, M. E., Fendrich, M., Libby, S., Goldenberg, D. & Grossman, J. (1996), Assessment of knowledge gains in proactive training for postvention. *Suicide and Life-Threatening Behav.*, 26:161–174.

Martin, G., Kuller, N. & Hazell, P. (1992), The effect on adolescents of the completed suicide of another student. *Youth Studies Australia*, 11:21–23.

Mattison, R. E. (1993a), Consultation in the school environment. In: *Child and Adolescent Mental Health Consultation in Hospitals, Schools, and Courts*, ed. G. K. Fritz, R. E. Mattison, B. Nurcombe & A. Spirito. Washington, DC: American Psychiatric Press, pp. 95–108.

————— (1993b), Principles in common school case consultations. In: *Child and Adolescent Mental Health Consultation in Hospitals, Schools, and Courts*, ed. G. K. Fritz, R. E. Mattison, B. Nurcombe & A. Spirito. Washington, DC: American Psychiatric Press, pp. 131–159.

————— & Spirito, A. (1993), Current consultation needs of school systems. In: *Child and Adolescent Mental Health Consultation in Hospitals, Schools, and Courts*, ed. G. K. Fritz, R. E. Mattison, B. Nurcombe & A. Spirito. Washington, DC: American Psychiatric Press, pp. 161–183.

Mauk, G. W., Gibson, D. G. & Rodgers, P. R. (1994), Suicide postvention with adolescents: School consultation practices and issues. *Educ. & Treatment of Children*, 17:468–483.

————— & Rodgers, P. R. (1994), Building bridges over troubled waters: School-based postvention with adolescent survivors of peer suicide. *Crisis Intervention & Time-Limited Treatment*, 1:103–123.

————— & Sharpnack, J. D. (1997), Grief. In: *Children's Needs II: Psychological Perspectives*, ed. G. G. Bear, K. M. Minke & A. Thomas. Bethesda, MD: National Association of School Psychologists, pp. 375–385.

————— & Weber, C. (1991), Peer survivors of adolescent suicide: Perspectives on grieving and postvention. *J. Adoles. Res.*, 6:113–131.

McEvoy, M. L. & McEvoy, A. W. (1994), *Preventing Youth Suicide*. Holmes Beach, FL: Learning Publications.

Moore, M. M. & Freeman, S. J. (1995), Counseling survivors of suicide: Implications for group postvention. *J. for Specialists in Group Work*, 20:40–47.

Morganett, R. S. (1990), *Skills for Living*. Champaign, IL: Research Press.

Oates, M. D. (1993), *Death in the School Community*. Alexandria, VA: American Association for Counseling and Development.

Parkes, C. M. (1988), Bereavement as a psychosocial transition: Processes of adaptation to change. *J. Social Issues*, 44(3):53–65.

Paul, K. (1995), The development process of a community postvention protocol. In: *The Impact of Suicide*, ed. B. L. Mishara. New York: Springer, pp. 64–72.

Peck, M. L. & Berkovitz, I. H. (1987), Youth suicide: The role of school consultation. *Adoles. Psychiat.*, 14:511–521.

Petersen, S. & Straub, R. L. (1992), *School Crisis Survival Guide*. West Nyack, NY: Center for Applied Research in Education.

Philip, A. F. (1990), Suicide and suicidal behavior: Postvention—Counseling center response. *J. College Student Psychother.*, 4:195–209.

Pitcher, G. D. & Poland, S. (1992), *Crisis Intervention in the Schools.* New York: Guilford.

Poland, S. (1989), *Suicide Intervention in the Schools.* New York: Guilford.

——— (1995), Best practices in suicide intervention. In: *Best Practices in School Psychology-III*, ed. A. Thomas & J. Grimes. Washington, DC: National Association of School Psychologists, pp. 459–468.

——— Pitcher, G. & Lazarus, P. J. (1995), Best practices in crisis intervention. In: *Best Practices in School Psychology-III*, ed. A. Thomas & J. Grimes. Washington, DC: National Association of School Psychologists, pp. 445–458.

Pynoos, R. S. & Nader, K. (1990), Mental health disturbances in children exposed to disaster: Preventive intervention strategies. In: *Preventing Mental Health Disturbances in Childhood*, ed. S. E. Goldston, J. Yager, C. M. Heinecke & R. S. Pynoos. Washington, DC: American Psychiatric Press, pp. 211–234.

Raphael, B. (1983), *The Anatomy of Bereavement.* New York: Basic.

Renaud, C. (1995), Bereavement after suicide: A model for support groups. In: *The Impact of Suicide*, ed. B. L. Mishara. New York: Springer, pp. 52–63.

Richardson, V. E. (1995), Crisis intervention in contemporary society: Contributions from critical theory. *Crisis Intervention & Time-Limited Treatment*, 1:177–189.

Roberts, W. B., Jr. (1995), Postvention and psychological autopsy in the suicide of a 14-year-old public school student. *School Counselor*, 42:322–330.

Ruof, S. R. & Harris, J. M. (1988), Suicide contagion: Guilt and modeling. *NASP Communique*, 16:8.

——— ——— & Robbie, M. B. (1987), *Handbook: Suicide Prevention in the Schools.* La Salle, CO: Weld Board of Cooperative Educational Services.

Sandoval, J. & Brock, S. E. (1996), The school psychologist's role in suicide prevention. *School Psychol. Quart.*, 11:169–185.

Schonfeld, D. J. (1993), School-based crisis intervention services for adolescents: Position paper of the Committees on Adolescent and School Health, Connecticut chapter of the American Academy of Pediatrics. *Pediatrics*, 91:656–657.

———— Kline, M. & Members of the Crisis Intervention Committee (1994). School-based crisis intervention: An organizational model. *Crisis Intervention & Time-Limited Treatment*, 1:155–166.

Schwab, R. (1986), Support groups for the bereaved. *J. for Specialists in Group Work*, 11:100–106.

Slaikeu, K. A. (1990), *Crisis Intervention*. Boston: Allyn & Bacon.

Smith, J. & Garza, L. (1989), *Project SOAR: Suicide, Options, Awareness, and Relief*. Dallas, TX: Dallas Independent School District.

Steele, W. (1992), *Traumatic and Troubling Losses for Children*. Detroit, MI: Institute for Trauma & Loss.

Tanney, B. (1995), After a suicide: A helper's handbook. In: *The Impact of Suicide*, ed. B. L. Mishara. New York: Springer, pp. 100–120.

Tedeschi, R. G. & Calhoun, L. G. (1993), Using the support group to respond to the isolation of bereavement. *J. Mental Health Counsel.*, 15(1):47–54.

Trachta, A. M. (1988), Postvention: Helping students deal with death. *Psychiatric Hosp.*, 19:165–168.

Turner, J. (1996), *Grief at School*. Washington, DC: American Hospice Foundation.

Valente, S. M. & Saunders, J. M. (1993), Adolescent grief after suicide. *Crisis*, 14(1):16–22, 46.

Wenckstern, S. & Leenaars, A. A. (1993), Trauma and suicide in our schools. *Death Studies*, 17:151–171.

Wrobleski, A. (1984), The suicide survivor's grief group. *Omega: J. Death & Dying*, 15:173–183.

Zimpfer, D. G. (1991), Groups for grief and survivorship after bereavement: A review. *J. for Specialists in Group Work*, 16:46–55.

Zinner, E. S. (1987), Responding to suicide in schools: A case study in loss intervention and group survivorship. *J. Counsel. & Develop.*, 65:499–501.

Note: The material and ideas in Table 1 were gleaned from the following sources: American Association of Suicidology (1997); Berman and Jobes (1991); Blom et al. (1991); Bozigar et al. (1993); Brock et al. (1996); Capuzzi (1994); Carter and Brooks (1990, 1991); Catone and Schatz (1991); Celotta (1995); Deaton and Berkan (1995); Dunne-Maxim et al. (1992); Grossman et al. (1995); Hazell (1991); Hicks (1990); Hundley and Bratton (1994); Komar (1994); Mauk and Rodgers (1994); Mauk and Weber (1991); Mauk et al. (1994); McEvoy and McEvoy (1994); Paul (1995); Petersen and Straub (1992); Pitcher and Poland (1992); Poland (1989, 1995); Poland et al. (1995); Renaud (1995); Roberts (1995); Ruof and Harris (1988); Ruof et al. (1987); Sandoval and Brock (1996); Schonfeld (1993); Schonfeld et al. (1994); Slaikeu (1990); Zinner (1987).

11 A PROGRAM OF COMPREHENSIVE SCHOOL-BASED MENTAL HEALTH SERVICES IN A LARGE URBAN PUBLIC SCHOOL DISTRICT: THE DALLAS MODEL

GLEN PEARSON, JENNI JENNINGS, AND JAMES NORCROSS

The long history of the relationship between adolescent psychiatry and public education is marked by a kind of reciprocal ambivalence, varying in intensity over time, from mutual neglect to territorial conflict. Over the past 30 years, educators and psychiatrists as professional groups have experienced many changes in the scientific, social, legal, economic, and political environments in which each must carry out its mission. Psychiatry has weathered the community mental health and patient advocacy movements, a nosological revolution, an explosion of knowledge in neuroscience and psychopharmacology, the rise and fall of proprietary psychiatric hospitals, deinstitutionalization of the seriously and persistently mentally ill, and, not least of all, the headlong implementation of managed care currently under way. Public education has borne the brunt of the burden of regressive social anomie in our inner cities—poverty, racial conflict, high crime rates, alcoholism, drug addiction, and family and youth violence—while enduring unendingly shifting pressures for change, including such trends as site-based school management, school improvement modeling, mental health and substance abuse curricula, community services programs, and federally mandated special education services to disabled or handicapped children. Although psychiatrists and educators have always been invested in producing healthy, well-educated, productive citizens, both have usually been too preoccupied with the vicissitudes of their own professional domains to see the larger picture of their shared common purpose, let alone come together and work synergistically in its service.

207

In 1993, in response to a request by two school principals, Dallas's public mental health agency helped the school staff to initiate a collaborative mental health clinic using existing resources and personnel along with a child and adolescent psychiatrist. In the 5 years that followed, this model matured, developed, and grew into a district-wide program of health, comprehensive mental health, and youth and family services in 10 sites serving all 160,000 students in more than 200 schools. In this chapter, we review the literature on school-based mental health services, trace the development of the Dallas service delivery model to its present configuration, and report the results of its program evaluation. We also discuss some of the advantages we have discovered, as well as the challenges that we have faced and those which still confront us.

Review of the Literature

Healthcare services have been provided in schools since the late 19th century, when doctors monitored outbreaks of infectious diseases such as tuberculosis and diphtheria. Even then, programs were plagued with funding problems, arguments over service responsibilities, and difficulty establishing and maintaining collaborative agreements (Dryfoos and Klerman, 1988). Although lacking in organization, services survived and even began to proliferate when the issue of teen pregnancy surfaced (Balassone, Bell, and Peterfreund, 1991). The social, psychological, and health problems of children necessitate a comprehensive approach (Halfon, Inkelas, and Wood, 1995). This has been especially true for teenagers, who have their own set of health issues due to risk-taking behaviors, difficulty accessing care, confidentiality, and the emotional upheaval that often characterizes adolescence (Brindis and Sanghvi, 1997). Schools have proved to be a vitally important site for the establishment of mental health services for children, as other existing community resources too often cannot meet this need (Flaherty, Weist, and Warner, 1996).

Historically, healthcare services and mental health services have been seen as separate and distinct—a dichotomy maintained over the years by such influences as the stigma associated with mental illness, the lack of hard medical evidence of the effectiveness of psychiatric treatment, the resistance of the profession to change, and financial barriers to accessing mental health services. Over the past 20 years, however, a revolution in neuroscience and the rapid development of effective biological therapies has helped reestablish the link between psychiatry and medicine. The partnering of health, mental health, and schools has brought about its own set of conflicts: turfism, funding issues, differences in eligibility for services, paperwork, accountability, and colocation issues (Hacker et al., 1994). Relationships between mental health providers and school personnel have often been awkward, even competitive, with differing ideologies regarding what is best for the child.

Successful integration of services requires interorganizational cooperation: interdependence, mutual benefit, common modes of communication, and complementary technologies (Goldman, 1982). Gottlieb and Kotch (1984) have suggested guidelines for developing school-based services: convening a network of partners, assessing healthcare needs and resources, deciding what services to offer, delineating gaps and duplications, choosing a site, and developing and monitoring implementation. A well-designed health services program, combined with comprehensive health education, can significantly advance the health of the nation's children.

Once services are in place, students, parents, and school staff must know of their existence. Walter et al. (1995) found that referral sources in a large urban school clinic system consisted of clinic outreach (48%), self-referral (44%), and school staff referral (8%). Despite efforts to spread information, knowledge of available services is sometimes lacking. Reasons for nonuse by students include lack of parental permission, feelings that the clinic would not be able to help them, concerns about confidentiality, and no knowledge that the services existed (Balassone et al., 1991); others have reported not being able to leave class for appointments (Keyl et al., 1996); still others have complained of a lack of communication among school, parents, and health providers regarding needs and services available to meet them (Fox, Rankin, and Salmon, 1991).

Students use school-based clinics to meet a variety of healthcare needs, ranging from basic health education and screening to chronic psychosocial problems, and school sites have evolved to meet the ever-changing challenges of the youth they serve. Igoe and Goodwin (1991) note that the school is a likely site to target such tasks as properly immunizing the nation's pediatric population. A majority of clinics provides an array of services, including assessment and referral, treatment of minor injuries, routine health screening, sports physicals, nutrition information, laboratory services, birth control and pregnancy information, and mental health services (Balassone et al., 1991). Ryan, Jones, and Weitzman (1996) have underscored the importance of these services with their finding that urban junior high school students who used the school-based clinics were more likely to be involved in risk-taking behaviors (e.g., unprotected sex, physical violence, and substance abuse) and were also performing more poorly academically.

Although school-based health services have been in place for almost a century, the integration of mental health services is relatively new (Flaherty et al., 1996). A wide range of estimates of the prevalence of mental health issues in the help-seeking student population has been reported. Balassone et al. (1991) have reported that the most frequent visits were for general illness and sports physicals, but 20% were for mental health services. Others have found that as many as 50% of clinic visits are for such nonmedical reasons as peer and family issues, emotional problems, and substance abuse (Adelman and Taylor, 1996). Many physical complaints have psychogenic origins, and the treatment of many other health problems is enhanced by mental health services. Whatever their stated reason for a clinic visit, students often have other physical and mental health needs (Harold and Harold, 1993). A survey of Texas school nurses found that a significant amount of time is spent caring for students with special health needs; chronic medical problems were foremost among these, but attention deficit hyperactivity disorder ranked second only to asthma as a reason for nursing involvement.

In a survey of Colorado school personnel, Goodwin, Goodwin, and Cantrill (1988) found that poor decision-making skills, poor self-image, inability to resolve interpersonal conflict, depression, and conduct problems were the principal unmet mental health needs of students. Elementary-age users of school mental health services were reported to have more critical life events, more signs of familial disruption, and more involvement in special services (Cowen, Weissberg, and Guare, 1984). Gaps in and duplications of services can be eliminated (Gottlieb and Kotch, 1984). Consumers using the school-based clinics are as economically disadvantaged and as psychiatrically impaired as community clinic users but do not have easy access to the community clinics (Armbruster, Gerstein, and Fallon, 1997). Most needed services can be provided on site (Walter et al., 1995), and students frequently make return visits to the clinic (Ryan et al., 1996).

School-based health centers are now providing care to high-risk youth who may not receive it elsewhere. These clinics are targeting many of the 1990 "Health Objectives for the Nation": general health screening, improved pregnancy outcomes for adolescent mothers, decreased substance abuse, better control of stress, less suicidal ideation, improved nutrition, and more immediate treatment of accidents and injuries (Dryfoos and Klerman, 1988).

School clinic users have greater access to needed services than their nonusing peers. They report high ratings of clinic staff and services (Balassone et al., 1991) and demonstrate a higher rate of utilization of services of all kinds. Student self-reports show a significant decline in rates of depression and significant improvement in self-concept (Weist et al., 1996). Nonusers of services are more socially withdrawn than peers who take advantage of services; they have more total absences and lower grades (Weist et al., 1995).

Although further studies monitoring the outcomes of these programs are certainly needed, the evidence already available clearly shows that the integration of health and mental health services through partnership with the schools can only improve our ability to provide care to the nation's youth.

Program Development

The first school-based mental health services in Dallas were established by voluntary agreement between two local campus principals and the Dallas Mental Health/Mental Retardation Center (MH/MRC), facilitated by school psychology personnel who mediated the relationship. One child psychiatrist and one adolescent psychiatrist from the MH/MRC medical staff provided one half-day of direct services and consultation per week and was allowed to partner with campus-based school personnel to form a team. The school had considerable resources that could be coopted to develop services: one full-time advanced nurse practitioner, two school psychologists, one social worker, one counselor, and one parent ombudsman. All of these educational professionals brought considerable enthusiasm and dedication to the development of a collaborative, multidisciplinary mental health treatment team under the leadership of the child/adolescent psychiatrist. The process of development was made possible by the full support of the founding principals and their staffs, and it was the principals and their assistant administrators who generated the majority of early referrals to the program.

Initially, four hours of psychiatrist time were scheduled each week, from 2:00 p.m. to 6:00 p.m., in order to afford the opportunity for in-classroom consultation as well as after-school and after-work family appointments. (This scheduling paradigm has stood the test of time and continues to be the model for utilization of psychiatrist time most desired by families and staff.) The MH/MRC's interest at this point was primarily heuristic, around issues of case finding, needs assessment, and experimental service delivery redesign, with particular emphasis on improving accessibility. Among the many important discoveries of this early phase in the program's evolution were the following: Children and families who would not seek services from a public mental health clinic will accept them gladly if they are offered in a familiar, user-friendly, close-to-home setting; accessibility for patients translates into productivity for providers (as appointment compliance rates approach 100%); although there continues to be a need for traditional school consultation, the crying need articulated by school staff and families is for direct treatment services; and there already exists within the public schools a wealth of social and clinical service resources that can be pulled together from within if only a broad-enough vision is applied from without, given administrative encouragement and support.

The experimental program involving the first two campuses was so successful that word spread rapidly throughout the district, resulting in an almost immediate demand for the establishment of similar services; within six months, the model had expanded to serving 14 campuses in six additional sites. During this early expansion, new service sites were implemented in the same entrepreneurial fashion that had characterized the first pilot: Interested principals and school communities approached either MH/MRC or the district employees who were working within the informal collaborative and offered space and other resources in exchange for psychiatric and social services. Subsequent expansion efforts were influenced by three factors that surfaced unexpectedly in the 1994–1995 school year: (a) The school district's Health and Human Services division became concerned about issues of equity if the informal collaboration were allowed to continue expanding entrepreneurially, driven by local campus demand; (b) a politically powerful group of local elected officials and business leaders, which had been attempting, unsuccessfully, to drive the development of a student support program (from the top down) for several years, noticed the successful emergence of the grass-roots, bottom-up services program and began maneuvering to get in front of and coopt it; and (c) the rapid expansion of the mental health service program resulted in its encountering the pioneering initiative of the Parkland Health and Hospital System, which had already established and maintained healthcare services within the Dallas Public Schools for more than 20 years. All three converging issues were resolved in a bold stroke by the school district, whose Health/Human Services administrator—herself a mental health professional, a respected advocate for children's mental health, and an established friend of the mental health provider community—moved to consolidate the informal collaborative with the business leaders' and elected officials' initiative, under the aegis of the school district, and invite both Parkland and Dallas MH/MRC as partners to provide services together, under the title of Youth and Family Centers (YFCs). The school district also was able to provide infrastructure funding for the project, including facilities, management, support, and supplies— allowing the provider partners to concentrate on their missions of health and mental health service delivery. The YFCs have operated under this paradigm for almost three years; only now, the partners are in the process of legally structuralizing their interrelationships with formal memoranda of agreement. The trade-off of price paid (loss of entrepreneurial spirit and local community control) for value received (broadness of reach and equity) is discussed later, in the "Advantages" and Challenges" sections.

Program Description: Dallas Youth and Family Centers

STRUCTURE

In the fall of 1993, two Dallas Public Schools campuses joined with Dallas MH/MRC and established the first intensive school-based mental health center. Within six months, the program expanded to 14 additional campuses. School-based centers experienced dramatic further growth until the fall of 1995, when Parkland Health and Hospital System, Dallas Public Schools, and Dallas MH/MRC formed a collaboration establishing the YFCs to provide integrated physical and mental health care in school-based settings.

UNIQUE PROGRAM FEATURES

Each of the 10 YFCs is geographically located to serve 20 to 25 school campuses. Each "family of schools" (Adelman and Taylor, 1996) includes a few high schools and all of their feeder elementary and middle schools. Each school campus provides a member of its student support team as liaison to the YFC in order to facilitate referral and implement the school service part of the child's treatment plan.

STAFFING

The school district employs a licensed mental health professional as YFC manager at each site. YFC managers lead and coordinate the activities of a team of health professionals from Parkland, a team of mental health professionals from Dallas MH/MRC, and several part-time school staff. Health team members include pediatricians, nurse practitioners, physician assistants, and social workers. Mental health professionals include child and adolescent psychiatrists, intake/assessment workers, and nonpsychiatric clinical service providers. School district employees who work part-time in the YFC programs include school psychologists, social workers, counselors, nurses, marriage and family therapists, and parent educators. Dallas MH/MRC provides 24-hour crisis response capability and physician on-call services.

TRAINING

Both pre-service and in-service training are integral parts of the YFC program. Predoctoral internships in psychology and social work are offered in collaboration with the graduate schools of several area universities. General psychiatry residents and child/adolescent psychiatry fellows at the University of Texas Southwestern Medical School are routinely assigned to rotations in the YFCs. Two semesters annually of child development training are provided to YFC staff members by volunteer faculty from the Dallas Psychoanalytic Institute, and all three partner agencies participate in a monthly school-based clinic grand rounds in which cases and current scientific topics are presented and discussed.

GUIDING PRINCIPLES

An integrated, holistic approach to addressing children's needs, particularly those of at-risk children, requires coordinated, family-focused, prevention-oriented, community-centered programming, developed in

214

response to the self-identified needs of local school communities. Some of the principles that inform the operation of YFCs are belief in a holistic approach to addressing children's developmental needs; belief in family-focused and prevention-oriented services; and beliefs that health and mental health services should be available to all children and families, that schools play a central role in the lives of children and adolescents, that a child's well-being affects his or her academic performance, and that all families have strengths and resources and must be empowered to participate in their children's education, growth, and development. It is our intent that every aspect of our program should reflect these beliefs.

The YFC partners believe that valuing and empowering families and friends produces positive changes for the school and community and creates opportunities for parents and families to participate fully in their children's education.

SERVICE DELIVERY PROCESS

Referral

Referrals to the YFCs are initiated by several sources: parents, school staff, and community agencies. School student support teams (SSTs), trained by YFC staff, screen student referrals and request YFC services in one or more of five major components: intensive mental health care, physical health care, counseling, family/home involvement, and youth development activities.

The major student referral categories for intensive mental health services are behavioral/emotional issues, family/home issues, and delinquent behavior. Behavioral issues include such symptoms as hyperactivity, impulsivity, aggressive behavior, conflict with teachers, and peer relationship difficulties; emotional issues include depression, anxiety, social withdrawal, and somatic complaints; family/home referrals may reflect issues relating to divorce, separation, marital conflict, abuse, or neglect; and referrals for delinquent behavior are characterized by truancy, stealing, assault, or gang involvement.

Service Prototype

The YFC program provides a collaborative multidisciplinary mental health treatment team, co-led by the child and adolescent psychiatrist and the YFC manager (licensed mental health professional). The team approach is reflected in every phase of service delivery: intake, evaluation/assessment, treatment, and follow-up. Concomitant with the multidisciplinary professional teamwork, the school staff participates in the child-centered plan of treatment and related service, which is developed and implemented across the contexts of school, home, and community; successful outcomes depend on the involvement of adults in all these sectors who touch the students' lives.

Upon enrollment in a YFC, a child can expect to receive services throughout his or her school life, from preschool through Grade 12. School success indicators for each student are tracked each school year, and aggregate data on these indicators are reported as feedback to YFC staff and sponsoring partner agency administrators and boards of trustees.

YFCs are open 5 days a week, with extended evening hours (until 8 or 9 p.m.) available Monday through Thursday. Twenty-four-hour, 7-day backup crisis services including emergency room and hospital care are provided by Parkland and Dallas MH/MRC.

Procedures

Mental health service delivery occurs in several steps, with full family participation expected throughout the process.

Step 1. The school campus SST compiles school data (records of grades, attendance, disciplinary referrals, special education services) on the referred student. The SST member interviews the student and family, observes the student in class, completes the Teacher Report Form of the Child Behavior Check List (CBCL; Achenbach and Edelbrock, 1986), and obtains parent permission for the child to receive YFC services. The compiled student data are forwarded to the YFC with a one-page summary referral form. Frequently, the school's campus liaison will consult with the YFC manager about the referred student.

Step 2. The family makes its first visit to the YFC, where intake staff complete initial assessment and paperwork (required by state funding authorities as part of program evaluation and performance contracting). Intake staff and site-based mental health professionals establish a relationship with the family and begin formulating the case for presentation to the collaborative evaluation team.

216

Step 3. The next step in service delivery is the collaborative team evaluation at the YFC. Team members always include the child and adolescent psychiatrist, the YFC manager, and such other mental health professionals and school staff members as are indicated by the circumstances. School staff, sometimes including classroom teachers and administrators, are often present; most referrals for mental health care are from school personnel, and the team values their direct participation. The YFC manager presents the case summary to the psychiatrist and team before the referred student and family join the group to be interviewed by the psychiatrist. Data from the interview are combined with observations from school and data from such instruments as the CBCL (parent, teacher, and youth self-report forms), and others required by the Texas Uniform Assessment, to arrive at a preliminary diagnosis, case formulation, and treatment plan.

A basic tenet of the model is the participation of all family members in the assessment and treatment processes: Grandparents and other extended family members often come to the table with their concerns, resources, and recommendations. The voices and visions of family members are highly valued; very often, families find immediate solutions to some of their most pressing problems.

Step 4. Treatment planning occurs at the conclusion of the team evaluation and takes advantage of having all the relevant members of the child's interlocking systems of family and school present for the process. The emphasis is on being comprehensive and on providing consistent interventions across systems while remaining problem oriented and solution focused. Specific strategies are detailed for both home and school (school service plan).

Step 5. Feedback to the referring school includes a copy of the school service plan, which is sent to the campus liaison at the referring school for implementation and monitoring. Each campus principal signs a contract at the beginning of the school year agreeing to work with the treatment team on recommended interventions.

Step 6. Therapeutic interventions are provided by mental health staff from both Dallas Public Schools and the Dallas MH/MRC. Providers include the psychiatrist, psychologists, social workers, licensed professional counselors, and rehabilitation skills trainers. Therapeutic modalities include individual therapy, group therapy, family therapy, play therapy, and adjunctive psychopharmacology. Bilingual (Spanish/English) services are available. The principles guiding these therapeutic approaches are eclectic and practical, with a predominance of family-systems, psychodynamic, cognitive-behavioral, and interpersonal orientations. School intervention plans often include behavior management plans, further psychometric evaluation, schedule or classroom assignment changes, mediation to resolve teacher–student conflict, and youth development activities. Interventions for the family to carry out at home are also a part of the treatment plan.

Step 7. Follow-up evaluation and treatment plan revisions are completed regularly (30 to 90 days) depending on the needs of each student and family. (The Texas Uniform Assessment requires a complete reassessment every 90 days regardless of the needs of the student.)

PROGRAM EVALUATION

The YFC program is evaluated annually by the Division of Research, Evaluation, and Information Systems of the Dallas Public Schools. Context, process, and outcome evaluation information is included in an annual report, the purpose of which is to review what services are provided, how the program is implemented, and the relationship between services and school success outcome measures. Context evaluation questions center on program goals and priorities, data from the project partners, and a review of literature concerning school-based mental and physical healthcare. Process evaluation questions address how the program is implemented, what quality assurances are in place, and how staff training addresses program needs. Outcome evaluation questions concern customer satisfaction and student school success outcomes (grades, attendance, behavior). Evaluation methodologies include interviews, questionnaires, follow-up data, attendance and discipline referral data, and student grades. Texas MH/MRC program evaluation data are collected and reported separately from the district's program evaluation; in addition to satisfaction and school success data, the MH/MRC program evaluation reports CBCL score changes, arrest rates, and certain "critical incident" occurrence rates (e.g., running away, placement outside the home).

Program Results

The staff at each YFC enters demographic information, presenting problems, and services received into the database during the traditional

66% male, 34% female
43% African-American, 38% Hispanic, 18% Anglo, 1% Asian
21% Siblings received services
68% Met poverty guidelines
60% At-risk for dropping out of school
27% Speakers of other Languages
24% Special Education
73% Free or reduced lunch
 4% Talented and gifted
34% PK-3, 24% 4-6, 19% 7-8, 23% 9-12

Figure 1 Student/family demographics (n = 1662).

school year (August–May). Results reported here are based on the 1996–1997 school year.

SAMPLE CHARACTERISTICS AND INTERVENTIONS

Student and family demographics are shown in Figure 1. One thousand six hundred sixty-two students and their families received intensive mental health services during the school year. The majority of the students were eligible for free or reduced-fee lunch (73%), met poverty guidelines (68%), and were considered at risk for dropping out of school (60%). Additionally, 27% were speakers of other languages, 24% were in special education, and 4% were in special programs for talented and gifted students. The patient group was 66% male, 43% African American, 38% Hispanic, 18% Anglo, and 1% Asian American. Information related to parents' employment status was collected for

819 families and is reported in Figure 2. Data suggest that these children were from families of working poor, with 79.8% reporting an employed parent or guardian versus 20.2% with no employed parent or guardian. Additionally, 21.7% reported both parents working. Information bearing on family type is summarized in Figure 3. Of the 1,100 families reporting, 42.4% were single-parent, 30.8% were nuclear, 13.3% were blended/married, 8.3% were multigenerational, 2.5% were blended/ unmarried, and 2.7% were of unspecified family type. Finally, as demonstrated in Figure 4, our families were overwhelmingly lacking in private health insurance (97% uninsured).

Presenting problems are summarized in Figure 5. Behavior problems comprised the majority of referral issues (66.4%); 20.2% were referred for emotional problems, 7.5% for family issues, 3.5% for academic problems, and 2.3% for "other" problems. Grade levels of referred students are shown in Figure 6; the referral rates for prekindergarten to Grade 3 (34%), Grade 4 to Grade 6 (24%), Grades 7 and 8 (19%), and Grade 9 to Grade 12 (24%) bear an uncertain relationship to theoretical developmental and academic transition phases, which are the focus of further study and consideration.

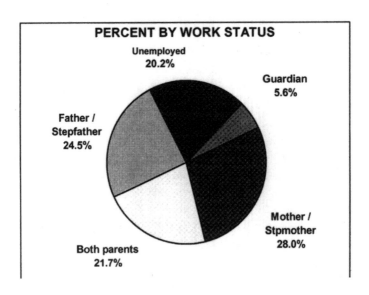

Figure 2 School-based mental health services.

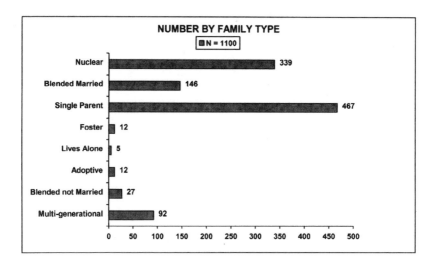

Figure 3 School-based mental health services.

Diagnostic Groups

The official diagnoses our patients have been given since the program opened in 1993 fall into seven general categories, summarized in Figure 7. The most common diagnoses have been disruptive behavior disorders (37%) and mood disorders (22%). Other diagnoses are adjustment disorders (14%), anxiety disorders (9%), personality disorders (7%), and V-codes (8%), with 2% unspecified or unknown.

An interesting finding is that, although school staff have a high index of suspicion for disruptive behavior disorders and overwhelmingly list behavior problems (66%) as the presenting problem, after evaluation only about half of the behavior problem children are diagnosed with disruptive behavior disorders. Many cases of apparently disruptive behavior are due to mood, anxiety, or adjustment disorders or to a nonpsychopathological disturbance in significant relationships in family or community.

Primary therapeutic interventions are summarized in Figure 8. Family therapy is the first-line intervention for 42.8% of referred cases. Other treatments include individual psychotherapy (30.9%), school interventions (13.7%), parent training (7.2%), support group (3%), group ther-

221

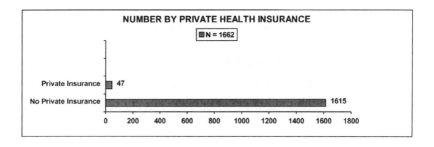

Figure 4 School-based mental health services.

apy (2.1%), and other or unspecified intervention (2%). Frequently, the treatments are combined in order to maximize therapeutic effects and to give extra support to the child and family or to the school staff. Prescription of psychopharmacological agents (Figure 9) occurred in 22% of the cases. Medication is never a primary therapeutic intervention; it is always considered an adjunct to one or more of the other modalities.

As previously noted in our guiding principles, all facets (home, school, community) of a child's environment influence his or her well-being (mental health, school performance, physical health); therefore, interventions are always provided across the contexts of home, school, and community.

OUTCOMES

Student Performance Outcomes

Data related to student attendance, grades, and behavior were compiled as baseline in the first or second 6-week term and as posttest follow-up in the sixth or final 6-week term of each of the 2 school years of the evaluation (1995–1996 and 1996–1997). There were fewer absences, course failures, and disciplinary referrals for both school years. Figure 10 shows a summary of results for the 1996–1997 school year. For mental health care, these improvements reflected as much as a 32% decrease in absences, a 31% decrease in course failures, and a 95% decrease in disciplinary referrals. The independent evaluator

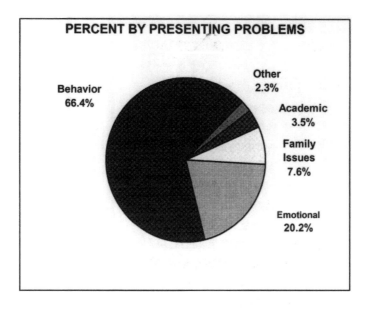

Figure 5 School-based mental health services.

concluded that effects in all three outcome measures were significant (Bush, 1997), with students who received intensive mental health intervention showing "meaningful decreases" in absences, course failures, and disciplinary referrals.

Student, Family, and School Personnel Satisfaction

Consumer questionnaires were completed by students and family members who received mental health care, and similar questionnaires were completed by school personnel who referred students to the YFCs. Family outcomes were positive, with an excess of 90% reporting that they were involved in their child's evaluation and treatment, that they would return to YFC for services, and that they were happy with the amount of time spent with them and how they were treated by staff. Student satisfaction was similarly high, with more than 90% reporting satisfaction with the amount of time spent and how they were treated, 90% reporting that they were doing better or much better since they received services, and 80% reporting that their families were doing better or much better since the intervention. As for school personnel,

223

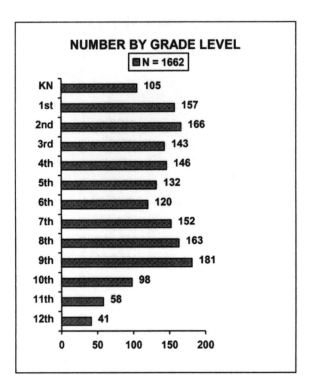

Figure 6 School-based mental health services.

more than 95% reported being satisfied with services. Similarly, high percentages described the services as being of high quality and said that they would recommend YFC services to other schools (Bush, 1996, 1997).

Discussion

What have we learned from our first 5 years of experience providing community mental health services on site in the public schools? That this service delivery model brings many advantages for patients, families, schools, and service providers is now nearly axiomatic; it is also true that attempts to establish and maintain such a service delivery system face many arduous challenges.

Number and Percentage of MHMR Initial Visits by Diagnosis		
Disruptive Behavior Disorders	254	37.2%
Mood Disorders	153	22.4%
Anxiety Disorders	60	8.8%
Adjustment Disorders	99	14.5%
Personality Disorders	46	6.7%
V- Codes	57	8.3%
Other	14	2.1%
TOTAL	683	100.%

Figure 7 School-based mental health services.

ADVANTAGES

For children and families, the advantages of the school-based model are obvious: Services are close to home, accessible, user friendly, and relatively devoid of stigma. For providers and school staff, it is very gratifying to be able to work with and effect change in some of the most crucial environmental variables that affect the child's functioning (home, school, community); community service providers in traditional models of service delivery have been long accustomed to seeing only a fraction of their appointed clinical service hours, owing to high noncompliance rates; compliance rates approaching 100% are not unheard of in school-based settings. For agency administrators, the most important finding is that improved accessibility for consumers translates directly into vastly improved productivity of agency provider staff. If we take our services to where the kids are, rather than give the kids appointments to come see us, we will experience a great deal less downtime in general and will be helpful to many who otherwise would never have sought our services.

CHALLENGES

As the model has expanded and matured, we have begun to notice that appointment compliance rates, which were initially extremely high,

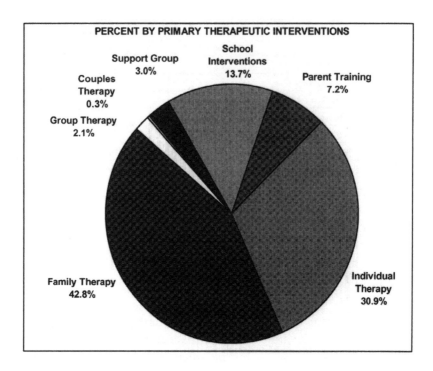

PERCENT BY PRIMARY THERAPEUTIC INTERVENTIONS

Figure 8 School-based mental health services.

are declining in school-based sites. We attribute this to a kind of satiation in the target population: Now that we are more accessible (but not nearly accessible enough, with each site serving 20 to 25 school campuses), the same public mental health client mentality that pervades our own outpatient clinics has infected our outreach centers. This is a particularly worrisome trend, as mental health agency adminis-trators attempt to plan further allocation of scarce resources in the community.

Political and territorial boundary issues are formidable challenges for a collaboration such as ours. From the beginning, our operational partners have shared a common vision and purpose; we have respected one another and supported one anothers' missions. During the same period of time, each of our sponsoring governing bodies has experienced severe political vicissitudes of one kind or another, some of which could have been life-threatening to our nascent collaboration—the

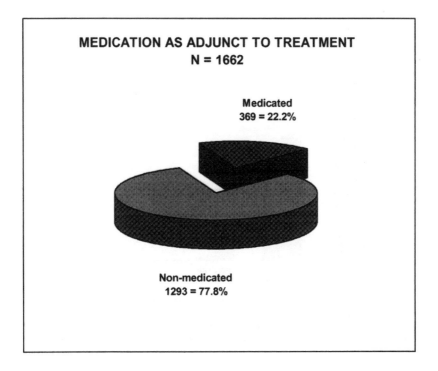

MEDICATION AS ADJUNCT TO TREATMENT
N = 1662

Medicated
369 = 22.2%

Non-medicated
1293 = 77.8%

Figure 9 School-based mental health services.

school's board of trustees hiring and firing a superintendent and engaging in internecine warfare; the mental health board of trustees hiring and firing an executive director and trying to micromanage YFC operations, until brought up short by a State Auditor's Office investigation; and the hospital district's board getting involved in the controversy over the provision of family planning and reproductive healthcare services to adolescents. The providers of clinical and social services to youth, represented by the operational arms of all three agencies, have clung to their mutual respect and support for one another through it all, but maintaining services in such an uncertain and heated political climate remains a questionable proposition.

The advent of managed care in the provision of both healthcare and behavioral healthcare services hangs heavy over all three partners in our enterprise. We are all significant providers of Medicaid-funded services, albeit under differing Medicaid "program options." Hereto-

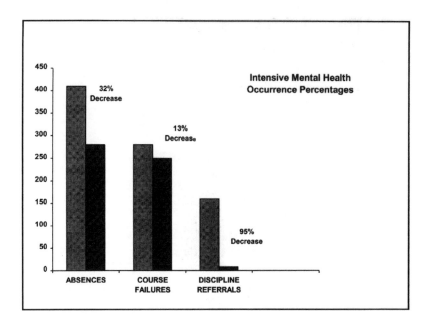

Figure 10 School-based mental health services: Student success outcomes 1996–1997.

fore, the Dallas MH/MRC has been an exclusive provider of rehabilitation option program services; Dallas Public Schools has been the provider of school health and related services, and Parkland has been the provider of early prevention, screening, diagnosis, and treatment services. Under a pending plan by the state of Texas to modify the provision of healthcare and behavioral healthcare services under a new Medicaid 1915(b) waiver, Dallas County and six surrounding counties will come under the supervision of a yet-to-be-appointed local behavioral healthcare authority, which will supervise the administration of services, delivered by competitively secured managed behavioral healthcare organizations (which may or may not include our existing community mental health centers). Under these conditions, our two provider partners must be concerned not only about retaining "market share" but, indeed, about survival. An interesting leitmotif in the prevailing maneuvering among the agencies is the loyalty of the operational divisions of our partners to one another, even as the superordinate organizations compete and, potentially, clash.

Conclusion

Providing integrated health and mental health services in the public schools has advantages for all the stakeholder groups: children and families, school authorities, providers of clinical services, and public agency administrators. Vastly improved accessibility for consumers translates into enhanced productivity for treatment providers. The outcomes of school-based mental health services are promising in terms of clinical symptom reduction, school success indicators, and stakeholder satisfaction.

A multidisciplinary, multiagency interprofessional team approach to service delivery is an effective way of integrating diverse resources and bringing them to bear upon the mental health problems of children and families. Psychiatrists have a key role as leader of the clinical team, provider of psychiatric services, and clinical supervisor of other mental health professionals on the team. The confluence of several current trends in public education and psychiatry makes the present a time ripe with opportunities for collaboration to improve the mental health of our children and their families.

REFERENCES

Achenbach, T. M. & Edelbrock, C. S. (1986), *Manual for the Teacher Version of the Child Behavior Checklist and Revised Child Behavior Profile*. Burlington, VT: Author.

Adelman, H. S. & Taylor, L. (1996), Addressing barriers to learning: Beyond school-linked services and full service schools. *Amer. J. Orthopsychiat.*, 67:408–421.

Armbruster, P., Gerstein, S. H. & Fallon, T. (1997), Bridging the gap between service need and service utilization: A school-based mental health program. *Community Mental Health J.*, 33:199–211.

Balassone, M. L., Bell, M. & Peterfreund, N. (1991), A comparison of users and non-users of a school-based health and mental health clinic. *J. Adoles. Health*, 12:240–246.

Brindis, C. D. & Sanghvi, R. V. (1997), School-based health clinics: Remaining viable in a changing health care delivery system. *Annual Rev. Public Health*, 18:567–587.

Bush, J. (1996), *Final Evaluation Report of the 1995–1996 Youth and Family Centers. Title XI (REIS96-350-2)*. Dallas, TX: Dallas Public Schools, Division of Research, Planning, and Evaluation.

———— (1997), *Final Evaluation Report of the 1996–1997 Youth and Family Centers: Title XI (REIS97-350-2)*. Dallas, TX: Dallas Public Schools, Division of Research, Planning, and Evaluation.

Cowen, E. L., Weissberg, R. P. & Guare, J. (1984), Differentiating attributes of children referred to a school mental health program. *J. Abnorm. Child Psychol.*, 12:397–409.

Dryfoos, J. G. & Klerman, L. V. (1988), School-based clinics: Their role in helping students meet the 1990 objectives. *Health Educ. Quart.*, 15:71–80.

Flaherty, L. T., Weist, M. D. & Warner, B. S. (1996), School-based mental health services in the United States: History, current models and needs. *Community Mental Health J.*, 32:341–352.

Fox, T. K., Rankin, M. G. & Salmon, S. S. (1991), How schools perceive the school health service. *Public Health*, 105:399–403.

Goldman, H. H. (1982), Integrating health and mental health services: Historical obstacles and opportunities. *Amer. J. Psychiat.*, 139:616–620.

Goodwin, L. D., Goodwin W. L. & Cantrill, J. L. (1988), The mental health needs of elementary schoolchildren. *J. School Health*, 58:282–287.

Gottlieb, N. H. & Kotch, J. R. (1984), Maximizing school health services in a time of fiscal restraint. *J. School Health*, 54:27–29.

Hacker, K., Fried, L. E., Bablouzian, L. & Roeber, J. (1994), A nationwide survey of school health services delivery in urban schools. *J. School Health*, 64:279–283.

Halfon, N., Inkelas, M. & Wood, D. (1995), Non-financial barriers to care for children and youth. *Annual Rev. Public Health*, 16, 447–472.

Harold, R. D. & Harold, N. B. (1993), School-based clinics: A response to the physical and mental health needs of adolescents. *Health Social Work*, 18:65–74.

Igoe, J. B. & Goodwin, L. D. (1991), Meeting the challenge of immunizing the nation's children. *Pediatr. Nursing*, 17:583–585.

Keyl, P. M., Hurtado, M. P., Barber, M. M. & Borton, J. (1996), School-based health centers: Students access, knowledge and use of services. *Arch. Pediatr. Adoles. Med.*, 150:175–180.

Ryan, S., Jones, M. & Weitzman, M. (1996), School-based health services. *Curr. Opin. Pediatr.*, 8:453–458.

Walter, H. J., Vaughn, R. D., Armstrong, B., Krakoff, R. Y., Tiezzi, L. & McCarthy, J. F. (1995), School-based health care for urban minority junior-high school students. *Archives of Pediatr. Adoles. Medicine*, 149:1221–1225.

Weist, M. D., Paskewitz, D. A., Warner, B. S. & Flaherty, L. T. (1996), Treatment outcome of school-based mental health services for urban teenagers. *Community Mental Health J.*, 33:199–211.

———— Proescher, E. L., Freedman, A. H., Paskewitz, D. A. & Flaherty, L. T. (1995), School-based health services for urban adolescents: psychological characteristics of clinic users vs. non-users. *J. Youth Adoles.*, 24:251–256.

12   THE CURRENT CRISIS IN PSYCHOTHERAPY

AT BOARDING SCHOOLS:

PROTECTING THE INTERESTS

OF THE CHILD AND OF THE SCHOOL

RICHARD M. GOTTLIEB

Despite considerable professional activity by therapists and consultants over the years, and despite the quite unique conditions for mental health work in this important area, surprisingly little has been written about psychotherapy in the special setting of boarding schools. Although only 6 years have passed since I first wrote about the requirements and rewards of boarding-school work (Gottlieb, 1991), a near-revolution has occurred, profoundly although silently affecting these schools, students, therapists, and families alike. These often invidious changes have for the most part followed in the choppy wake of the transition of our national health care system toward a managed-care model. Along with effecting changes in the financial organization of health and mental health, managed care has brought complementary changes in the kinds of treatments available and, perhaps most significantly, in the prevailing models of emotional illnesses on which professionals rely. Furthermore, in pursuit of reductions in mental health care costs, managed-care monitors have turned to less qualified (at times to unqualified or under-qualified, and undersupervised) practitioners. Not only has quality of care suffered as a result, but the very concept of expertise itself (experience, qualification) has been undermined.

I was asked to give the keynote address for the April 1997 meeting of the Independent Schools Health Association—a national organization of independent schools, their health care givers, faculty, and administrators—on the subject, "Psychotherapy in the Boarding-School Setting: Protecting the Interests of the Child and of the School." My response to this charge, which forms the basis of this chapter, was to question its premise. It seemed to me then, and it has continued to seem to me now, that the psychotherapeutic enterprise was under siege throughout our health care system. The boarding-school setting is no exception. It is perhaps an irony that the conditions for good, solid psychotherapeutic activity need protection every bit as much as the interests of child and school. Indeed, it is likely that the latter are vulnerable as long as the former lack protection.

For the past 23 years, I have worked with troubled students, consulted with troubled heads of schools about some very thorny issues, treated my share of faculty members and administrators, helped families not to interfere with the school's mission for their children, and participated in admissions processes, readmissions processes, and disciplinary and dismissal proceedings. I have—with great satisfaction—attended my share of graduation exercises during which students and families with whom I had become close celebrated their having made it to the end. We have prevailed against what sometimes seemed insurmountable odds. Such deep satisfactions are among the common rewards for those of us who have chosen to work as educators and helpers with children and adolescents.

Yet, great as such satisfactions can be, it troubles me to have to add that there are new tensions abroad in the greater society that threaten our capacity to carry on this work with spontaneity and creativity. There are enormous hidden costs of complying with the letter of the law, of living in a more litigious environment, and of avoiding trouble. If one risks trouble by being affectionate with a student, if it is difficult to define the line over which one may not safely step, then one answer is to withdraw from spontaneity, creativity, and passionate involvement in the job at hand. This withdrawal, safe though it may seem, represents a sterilization of our work: Very few teachers and other school personnel have pursued their careers as a way to avoid intense engagement with others. Most love this work precisely because of its engagement with others. How many of us would really bring our lawyer along on a date in order to avoid being charged with sexual harassment? And yet, isn't that what we are threatened with having to do in an atmosphere in which so much of our behavior seems potentially actionable?

We face a dilemma, and we need appropriate language to describe it. With constraints, intrusions, directives, and warnings impinging on our small world from the greater society, how can professionals respond without abandoning their missions or without losing track of the reasons why they have chosen this kind of work in the first place? How can educators comply with the legitimate claims of the outside world without becoming frightened into rigidity, emotional withdrawal, paralysis, indecision, apathy, or cynicism?

What Is "Protection," and Who Needs It?

The dictionary tells us that the verb *to protect* derives from a Latin word that means "to cover in front" or "to defend" (also "to cover over or from above" in the sense of providing a sheltering roof). We know from experience that psychotherapy requires protection for its effective conduct: protected space, protected time, protected communications, and protection for both participants from the immediate intrusions of the outside world and from each other. My experience has caused me deep concerns that psychotherapy in boarding schools has become increasingly difficult if not impossible and that—extreme as it may sound—if current trends continue, it is in danger of extinction.

The boarding-school setting has always presented its own special set of challenges to the therapeutic process. Our adolescent population has proved perennially difficult to engage in the "talking therapies." The uneven schedule of the boarding-school year has always made it difficult to establish and maintain the kind of regular, reliable schedule of meetings that promotes stability in a therapeutic relationship. The special developmental issues and tasks of the adolescent period, most centrally those having to do with the movement toward adult separateness and the emergence of adult sexuality, may make us feel more like observers than persons with much influence over process or outcome.

From its beginnings, the practice of psychotherapy was a very private affair. Privacy was a condition of helpfulness. In the therapeutic situation, a client or patient could unburden himself of his deepest, closely kept, shameful, guilt-ridden, embarrassing, or humiliating concerns without fear that his secrets would ever find their way out of the consulting room. The therapeutic relationship was once understood to require absolute confidentiality in order for the patient to bring to light those concerns that troubled him most. At the same time, it was a fundamental tenet of the theories of psychopathogenesis that these private thoughts and concerns lay at or close to the heart of each person's emotional troubles. It was understood that one's emotional symptoms had been caused, ultimately, by disturbances in the private sphere, be they of intimate sexuality or aggression. Emotional symptoms, it was held, were reflections of disturbances in desiring or hating. Consequently, for emotional healing to take place, these disturbances had to be communicated to another person, identified, and understood in new ways. Sometimes, the simple bringing to light of long-held shameful secrets had a therapeutic effect.

Over time, we have witnessed the steady erosion of what bit of privilege has remained. From the point of view of the patient or client, it has become less possible to experience the consultation room as a "safe place." Symmetrically, the therapy situation has become less safe for its practitioners as well.

What are the changes of which I speak?

- In general, we operate in a more litigious environment than we ever have, as school personnel, physicians, therapists, helpers, teachers, and so forth. No one is unaffected by the menacing shadow of a lawsuit, and this is especially so with respect to issues of sexual abuse and sexual harassment.
- In the name of cost containment, the unregulated and explosive growth of so-called managed-care health insurance has selectively promoted certain models of illness and treatment, severely narrowed treatment options, and contributed to making medical confidentiality largely a thing of the past.
- Psychiatric medications—especially those that treat mood disorders—are far more effective than ever before. Paradoxically, their sometimes startling effectiveness, in combination with other factors, has contributed to the erosion of a legitimate place for the practice of psychotherapy.

Our Increasingly Litigious Environment—Sexual Harassment

We need no proof of the recently heightened tensions surrounding sexual harassment. Nonetheless, let me cite a headline over a story in the *New York Times* (Lewin, 1997): "New guidelines on sexual harassment tell schools when a kiss is just a peck." According to the article, "to protect themselves from liability, many school districts have adopted tough sexual harassment policies that have made teachers nervous about any physical contact with students" (p. 8). To make matters more difficult, "the guidelines reiterate the Education Department's position that schools can be held liable for student-to-student harassment if school officials knew about . . . [it], did not respond adequately, or failed to take adequate steps to prevent it" (p. 8). Beyond the threat of legal action by the Department of Education is a threat that worries schools far more: private lawsuits brought by parents.

SOME CONSEQUENCES OF ALLEGATIONS OF SEXUAL MISCONDUCT

A few years ago, my medical malpractice insurance carrier attached a new rider to my policy. The rider explained that, as it always had in the past, the insurance company would pay for all claims arising from my professional work and that it would pay for my legal defense up to the limits of the policy. In other words, the combined amounts of all defense costs plus all damages would be paid in full up to the overall limits of the policy, at that time in the range of several millions of dollars. However, the new rider stated that any claims involving an allegation of sexual misconduct on my part would be paid only to the amount of $25,000 and that the costs of my legal defense against such claims plus the amount of the settlement, if any, would in no event exceed $25,000. In other words, should an allegation be made against me of sexual misconduct, my insurance protection would virtually disappear. And note that all it would take to invoke this reduction of coverage was an allegation—not a finding, judgment, or settlement—of sexual misconduct.

THE REQUIREMENT TO REPORT

Hearsay Concerning Sexual Abuse.   Not long ago, some young men who claimed to have been sexually victimized as younger boys by a teacher at a boarding school in my area initiated lawsuits against that teacher, the school itself, and others. One of those sued was a psychiatrist who was working for the school, being paid on a retainer basis to do evaluations and psychotherapy with students. In their suit, the young men claimed that the psychiatrist had learned during his therapeutic work with one of them about the teacher's sexual misbehavior, and yet, they alleged, the psychiatrist had not reported the problem to the authorities. The suit against the psychiatrist has only recently been dropped. Despite the ultimately favorable outcome for this psychiatrist, for years he had to conduct his affairs with this litigation continuously festering in the background. The many years of misery and apprehension, fearful preoccupation, and damage to his reputation cannot be undone.

Suspected Danger to Another. Many readers are familiar with the decision some years ago of a California court that held that a therapist had the absolute obligation to report to authorities and to any endangered person any knowledge he may have gained in the course of therapeutic work that a person was endangered, even if that person was endangered by that therapist's patient and even if that patient had confided his intentions to harm during the course of treatment. There are few therapists, I believe, who, if they were told in therapy that their patient intended after leaving the session to murder another, would have any hesitation in reporting what they had learned to the appropriate authority. But, what about one of our boarding-school teenage boys, riddled with thoughts of violent, sudden impulsive actions toward a fellow student, who has presented himself for treatment because he is frightened of his own thoughts? What about a young, single, depressed faculty member who comes specifically to treatment for his attraction to a female student and his inner struggle against acting on this impulse?

Suspected Physical or Violent Abuse of a Child—Or the Worry That Such Abuse is Imminent. A few years ago, following a school vacation, a young male student mentioned to me in passing during a therapy session that his mother had chased him all about their apartment before dinner one night recently with a sharply pointed kitchen knife. As he was safely back at the boarding school, I decided that I did not have to worry about his immediate safety. In my mind, however, was a great concern for his safety when the school year ended and when he was scheduled to return to live with his mother full-time for the summer. In my mind also was a New York state law that required me to report any suspected physical abuse or endangerment of a child. There were some unexpected wrinkles as well. First, this child was a strapping 17-year-old. The mother was smaller, slower, and weaker than her son. Second, this was a stratum of society from which—naively and, I am afraid, blinded by unsuspected class prejudice—I had not expected to see a case of violent abuse or endangerment. Yet, after the boy's return home for summer vacation, he again reported to me that his mother continued chasing him about their home, kitchen knife in hand. It was a danger I could no longer defer reporting, so, after informing both mother and son that I would be doing so, I contacted the Bureau of Child Protective Services (BOPS) and made my report.

The results, as far as I knew them, were twofold. First, as I had known with certainty would happen, the boy's mother forbade the continuation of his therapy. Second, the BOPS officer kept in contact with me for months thereafter, and it was clear that with that organization's supervision, the threat of violence in the home had abated. In this instance, the interests of the child were protected to the extent that he was removed from danger; the interests of his boarding school were likewise protected, as he returned to school that fall and was ultimately graduated. Nevertheless, his therapy would have to wait.

DEALING WITH PARENTAL DISAPPOINTMENT

Some years ago, the head of a nearby school asked me to evaluate the extent of the continuing suicide risk for a student who had very recently executed a serious attempt on his life that had put him into a deep coma for 48 hours. The head and I worked out an understanding that I would be working for the school and not for the family. In initiating my discussions with the student and his family, I stressed that I would be conducting an evaluation for the school and that, furthermore, the school—not the family—would be paying my fees. After a careful and extensive evaluation, I informed the head that, in my opinion, the risk of more suicidal behavior was significant. He decided that it would better serve the interests of both school and student to deny him readmission.

Upon learning of the decision, the family, especially the boy's father, was furious at me. He demanded to read a copy of my evaluation; he hired another psychiatrist, who "found" that the boy was not at any continuing risk of suicide ("I'd stake my reputation on it," the other psychiatrist told me); he threatened to sue the school for readmission; and he threatened to sue me for some unspecified form of professional malfeasance. As it turned out, both of the boy's parents wielded considerable power in the community. As the situation deteriorated further, his father began to harass me with lengthy midnight telephone calls to my answering machine (he did not have my home number), during which, in an intoxicated state, he would threaten me with unimaginable ruin.

SOME NAVIGATIONAL AIDS: KNOWLEDGE, CLARITY

Certainly, navigation of these tricky shoals can present challenges. Yet, by what stars can we guide ourselves and our charges to a safe and secure course? To begin with, there is no substitute for a thoroughgoing familiarity with the legal, ethical, and regulatory environments that form a framework for our activities. We must know, for example, who has potential access to our records, both legitimately and by accident, and we must compose and keep those records while remaining fully mindful of their possible eventual disposition. Explicit discussions about the means with which we pursue our work, for whom we are working and to what ends, who shall pay our fees, and whose interest we serve will go a long way toward heading off troubles, as in my example of the disappointed father.

I never undertake to evaluate or treat a boarding-school child without the express consent of—or better yet, without the request—of that child's parent(s) or guardian(s). Someone on a school's staff will frequently call and ask me to evaluate a student, prescribe medication, or perhaps even begin therapy. My response, without fail, is to have that person ask the parents to call me. I will add, "You may want to tell the child's parents the nature of your concerns and why you think consultation with me is advisable. You may want to tell the parents who I am and how I have worked with children from this school. But I will be able to begin to work with this student and his family only after the parents have asked me to do so." (Emergencies, of course, must temporarily be handled differently, but situations of such extreme urgency are very rare indeed.)

AVOIDING CONFLICTS OF INTEREST

I make it clear to parents how and what I charge for my services, and I make it clear that I do not work for the school. It is a ready assumption of many parents that I do work for the school, and, in fact, many therapists who do boarding-school work are salaried by the schools at which they consult, are kept on a retainer arrangement, or operate as a kind of one-man mini-prepaid health plan, mental managed-care plan, or mental health maintenance organization (HMO).

The reason for my preference is quite simple. By working for a student and his family, I avoid conflict of interest. Much as we may wish that it were different, the interests of the child (and his family) can be quite divergent from or even directly at odds with the perceived or real interests of the school.

In my view, retainer and HMO/managed-care arrangements pose an additional set of conflicts of interest. These are the conflicts inherent in all managed-care types of arrangements: They may pit the interests of the patient against the financial interests of the therapist or doctor. The doctor who has contracted with the school to provide all of its mental health services for a prearranged fee will have diminished incentive to take on a difficult and time-consuming therapy situation with the aim of keeping the child functioning at school while he recovers. Such arrangements will tend to foster hasty suspensions and dismissals from school, actions that may be in the best financial interest of the therapist but not of the student, his family, or necessarily the school.

Some Ill Effects of So-Called Managed Care

A nationwide revolution has been in progress in our systems for the delivery of health care. In the name of cost containment, the unregulated and explosive growth of so-called managed-care health insurance has selectively promoted new models of illness and treatment, severely narrowed treatment options, and made medical confidentiality largely a thing of the past.

Although it is true that some practitioners working with boarding schools are directly affected by managed-care affiliations, for the most part medical and psychotherapeutic care provided to our students still remains outside the reach of managed-care networks. As managed-care companies increase in size, our status as outsiders to this extremely problematic system will disappear. As this happens, our efforts to protect the interests of the child and the interests of the school will have competition from a new corner—the compulsion (often contractual) to protect the interests of the insurance company, its executives, and its stockholders.

The managed-care industry has succeeded in redefining many of the key concepts and operations on which effective psychotherapy has been based in the past. To an alarming extent, even without exerting a significant and direct financial influence on us in boarding-school environments, the managed-care revolution has changed what we do.

MANAGED CARE HAS EFFECTIVELY PROMOTED ONE OF SEVERAL MODELS OF ILLNESS AND TREATMENT

For many years, there have been two major competing models for understanding the causes and directing the treatment of emotional disturbances: the so-called biological model and the psychogenic model. Much of the battle between these has been fought with depression as the paradigmatic illness and medication versus psychotherapy as the competing treatment modalities. From a scientific point of view, the struggle for dominance has been a draw, with the most definitive studies concluding that treatment approaches that combine medication and psychotherapy are more effective than either approach used alone.

Enter managed care, which effectively separates the financial interests of "providers" from the best medical interests of policyholders. Medication, by far the cheaper treatment modality, carries the day. Therapists from all disciplines will tell you that referring the managed-care policyholder for medication treatment proceeds unimpeded, but, for that policyholder to be able to have psychotherapeutic treatment, every kind of obstacle must be confronted and overcome. This begins with the need to secure the insurer's "prior approval" for work with the patient in therapy. If approval is granted (i.e., psychotherapy is deemed "medically necessary" by the insurer), such approval is given for a few meetings only. The procedure must be repeated every few sessions; all the while, the continuity of the treatment hangs in the balance. Often, reporting a degree of improvement will render the future of the treatment bleak. Commonly, it is therapists' fatigue that brings the effort to a close.

For those working in the boarding-school environment, there is spillover. The illness and treatment models favored by managed-care companies have taken on an authority that generates pressure for unrealistically brief diagnostic evaluations and the too hasty prescription of medication.

CARE MANAGEMENT HAS IMPLICITLY OR EXPLICITLY SEVERELY NARROWED TREATMENT OPTIONS

The narrowing of treatment options follows logically. If the most advantageous way of conceptualizing the cause of illness is as biologic, genetic, or constitutional, it seems to follow (not necessarily logically!) that psychotropic medications provide the best and most effective treatments. Certainly, they are the least expensive. Pressures can be great on the managed-care provider not to explain to the patient that there are other, if more expensive, ways to treat his illness. Although we may finally be seeing the end of the so-called gag clauses in managed-care providers' contracts with insurers, each provider knows well that being a team player tends to maximize bonuses, minimize reimbursement "holdbacks," encourage more referrals, and ensure his continued membership on the team.

"MANAGED CARE" HAS CONTRIBUTED TO MAKING CONFIDENTIALITY LARGELY A THING OF THE PAST

There are many threats to the assurance of the confidentiality that is the lifeblood of the therapeutic enterprise. These arise from sources with varying degrees of legitimacy. One of the most legitimate is one we have to negotiate on nearly a daily basis in boarding schools. Because our charges are minors, our schools must often act in loco parentis. To act effectively in the place of the parents, we require information. Our students, being immature of judgment, may not make their own best decisions. In the psychotherapeutic treatment of children, the exchange of information between therapist and parents is necessarily a much freer affair than it can properly be in the treatment of adults. Our teenage population confronts us with more complexity. We must sometimes make a judgment call with respect to communicating our concerns about a teenager—still immature, but much less so than younger children—to his parents or to those serving in their place.

The managed-care environment views the problem of confidentiality from an entirely different angle. The principle seems to be that he who pays the bill has the unfettered right to know what goes on! There is no question here of the impaired judgment of the immature; there is no question of clear and present dangers to self and others; there is only intrusion "justified" by a financial interest. The anonymity promised to therapists and policyholders alike is beyond the capacity of the insurers to provide, even if promised in good faith.

If there is spillover here of importance to therapy in school settings, it lies in the devaluation of privacy, the cheapening of confidentiality, and the increasing vulnerability of the private sphere to intrusion and violation—trends discernible not only in the care-management business but in our society as a whole.

Some Paradoxes of the Newer, Powerful Psychiatric Medications

We have in recent years been the beneficiaries of some nearly miraculous developments in chemistry. The genie in our pharmacologic bottle has been set loose, fetching us a bounty of highly effective psychiatric medications. Foremost among these have been the so-called SSRIs (selective serotonin re-uptake inhibitors). These medicines have been found highly effective in relieving certain depressions and ameliorating symptoms in some people suffering the ravages of obsessive-compulsive disorder. They also seem to relieve some symptoms of panic anxiety, social inhibitions or shyness, lack of assertiveness, and even delusions in some people.

It seems a Faustian bargain that among the most frequent major side effects of this class of compounds is a loss or disturbance of sexual interest and function. Patients report that they have lost their sexual desire or libido, that they have become difficult to arouse, and that their performance is adversely affected. For men, erection may become impossible or unreliable.

Most often, the loss of sexual interest and function is unwelcome, so much so at times that a patient will find these drugs intolerable. This is all well known. I want, however, to discuss the issue of the use—and I believe overprescription—of these medications in our boarding-school populations. We must bear in mind that the effectiveness of the SSRIs in teenagers can be equivocal. But the main difficulty has precisely to do with these drugs' impact on sexual desire and functioning. In our special school population, libido occupies an absolutely central position. It would not be too much of an exaggeration to say that, for our teenagers, libido is the name of the game. What happens sexually during this developmental epoch is destined to be remembered and influential for a long time to come. It takes only a bit of imagination to begin to appreciate the developmental complications that can so easily be introduced into an already fragile situation, due to a medication that diminishes or ablates normal desire or that interferes with performance.

Against this background, it is difficult indeed to justify the casual prescription of these medications. Yet, the confluence of several factors can and do, in my experience, contribute to quick prescriptions for teenagers: their effectiveness in some situations; the now dominant model of illness and treatment; tendencies toward marginalization of the psychiatric profession to *DSM–IV* diagnosis and treatment with medication; and, finally, because asking a psychiatrist for a "medication evaluation" is one of the few—if not the only—remaining ways that a nonmedical therapist and colleague can request consultation, help, or supervision on a difficult case that is not going well.

Summary and Conclusions

I have turned the assignment a bit on its head. I have, I suspect, surprised you by directing your attention to the fact that psychotherapy is itself in urgent need of our protection. Only after we have ensured its increasingly imperiled place in the school community and the larger community we will be in a position to think clearly about the protection of its participants and its setting. How can we ensure that we will be able to carry on with this important work in the presence of an increasing array of threats and obstacles?

First, we must fully recognize the features of the terrain: the laws, the regulatory environment, requirements for oversight, administrative procedures, and the nature of the organizations and individuals with whom we interface. We must be prepared to be flexible and to negotiate. Second, we cannot forget that our accustomed way, though familiar and traditional, is neither infallible nor beyond the need for revision. Psychotherapy is not for everyone and not for every ill. Theories of emotional disturbance, like all theories, are subject to modification or outright discarding when they no longer fit the data.

Yet, excessive mindfulness of the intrusive elements is an encumbrance. I remind you again of the man who brought his lawyer along on a date for counsel regarding sexual harassment. If we become too frightened to touch, we are in danger of handling our charges with tongs. Students handled with tongs are as unlikely to prosper as are Harlow's infant monkeys raised by wire surrogate mothers. There is, of course, a balance to be struck, and, in a therapist, achieving the right balance is a delicate matter of constitution, training, experience, one's own therapy, and experiences in ongoing psychotherapy case supervision.

I have noticed over time that counselors do not regularly have access to experienced supervisors with whom to discuss their delicate and important work, and very rarely indeed is ongoing case supervision available. Yet, the nature and difficulty of the work cry out for the kind of supervision afforded psychotherapy trainees at all levels of development within graduate departments of clinical psychology, psychoanalytic institutes, medical school departments of psychiatry, and social work schools, to name but a few.

REFERENCES

Gottlieb, R. M. (1991), Boarding school consultation: Psychoanalytic perspectives. *Adolescent Psychiatry, 18*:180–197. Chicago: University of Chicago Press.

Lewin, T. (1997), New guidelines on sexual harassment tell schools when a kiss is just a peck. *The New York Times* (National Report Section), March 15, p. 8.

THE AUTHORS

E. JAMES ANTHONY, M.D. is Clinical Professor of Psychiatry and Human Behavior, George Washington University Medical School; Training and Supervising Analyst, Washington (D.C.) Psychoanalytic Institute; Consultant/Adolescent Psychiatrist, Chestnut Lodge Hospital, Rockville, Maryland; and past president, American Academy of Child and Adolescent Psychiatry.

AARON H. ESMAN, M.D. (editor) is Professor of Clinical Psychiatry (Emeritus), Cornell University Medical College, and Faculty, New York Psychoanalytic Institute.

GUNTER ESSER, PH.D. is Professor and Head, Department of Clinical Psychology, University of Potsdam, Germany.

RICHARD M. GOTTLIEB, M.D. is Associate Clinical Professor of Psychiatry, Albert Einstein College of Medicine and a member of the faculties of the New York Psychoanalytic Institute and the Psychoanalytic Institute of the New York University School of Medicine, New York City.

WOLFGANG IHLE is Clinical Psychologist, University of Potsdam, Germany.

STEVEN L. JAFFE, M.D. is Professor of Psychiatry, Emory University School of Medicine, Clinical Professor of Psychiatry, Morehouse University School of Medicine, and Director of Adolescent Substance Abuse Programs, Charter Peachford Hospital, Atlanta, Georgia.

JENNI JENNINGS, M.A. is Coordinator, Youth and Family Centers, Dallas (Texas) Public Schools.

PHILIP KATZ, M.D. is Professor of Psychiatry, University of Manitoba, Winnipeg, and a past president of the American Society for Adolescent Psychiatry.

STEVEN H. KATZ, PH.D. is Clinical Psychologist, Jewish Family Service, Seattle, Washington.

BARBARA LAY, PH.D. is Clinical Psychologist, Central Institute of Mental Health, Mannheim, Department of Child and Adolescent Psychiatry, Germany.

HOWARD D. LERNER, PH.D. is Clinical Assistant Professor of Psychology in Psychiatry, University of Michigan Medical School, Ann Arbor; and Faculty, Michigan Psychoanalytic Institute.

RICHARD MAROHN, M.D. (deceased) was Professor of Clinical Psychiatry, Northwestern University Medical School, Chicago, Illinois; a member of the faculty of the Chicago Institute for Psychoanalysis; and editor of *Adolescent Psychiatry.*

GARY W. MAUK, PH.D., NCSP is Senior Research and Evaluation Consultant, Spectrum Consulting, North Logan, Utah.

JAMES NORCROSS, M.D. is Associate Medical Director for Child and Adolescent Services, Dallas (Texas) Mental Health/ Mental Retardation Center; and Clinical Instructor of Psychiatry, University of Texas Southwestern Medical School, Dallas.

GLEN PEARSON, M.D. is Director, Child and Adolescent Services, Dallas Mental Health/Mental Retardation Center; and Clinical Professor of Psychiatry, University of Texas Southwestern Medical School, Dallas.

ELIZABETH PERL, PH.D. is Assistant Professor, Department of Psychiatry and Behavioral Sciences, Northwestern University Medical School, Chicago, Illinois, and is the author of a forthcoming book on psychotherapy with adolescent and young adult women.

DOMEENA C. RENSHAW, M.D. is Professor of Psychiatry and Director of the Sexual Dysfunction Clinic, Loyola University of Chicago.

MARTIN SCHMIDT, M.D. is Professor and Department Head, Clinic for Child and Adolescent Psychiatry and Psychotherapy, Central Institute for Mental Health, Mannheim, Germany.

JIM SHARPNACK, M.S. is a doctoral candidate in the Department of Psychology, Utah State University, Logan.

PHYLLIS TYSON, PH.D. is Associate Clinical Professor, Department of Psychiatry, University of California, San Diego, and Training and Supervising Analyst, San Diego Psychoanalytic Institute.

ALEX WEINTROB, M.D. is Clinical Associate Professor of Psychiatry, Cornell University Medical Center, New York City, and President, American Society for Adolescent Psychiatry, 1997–1998.

CONTENTS OF VOLUMES 1–22

Contents of Volumes 1–22

Contents of Volumes 1–22

Contents of Volumes 1–22

Index